I Just Haven't Met You Yet

Finding Empowerment in Dating, Love, and Life

TRACY STRAUSS

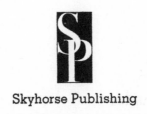

Skyhorse Publishing

Skyhorse Publishing books may be purchased in bulk at special discounts for sales promotion, corporate gifts, fund-raising, or educational purposes. Special editions can also be created to specifications. For details, contact the Special Sales Department, Skyhorse Publishing, 307 West 36th Street, 11th Floor, New York, NY 10018 or info@skyhorsepublishing.com.

Skyhorse® and Skyhorse Publishing® are registered trademarks of Skyhorse Publishing, Inc.®, a Delaware corporation.

Visit our website at www.skyhorsepublishing.com.

10 9 8 7 6 5 4 3 2 1

Library of Congress Cataloging-in-Publication Data is available on file.

Cover design by Paul Qualcom
Illustration by iStock

Print ISBN: 978-1-5107-4292-5
Ebook ISBN: 978-1-5107-4293-2

Printed in the United States of America

I might have to wait
I'll never give up
I guess it's half timing and the other half's luck . . .

—Michael Bublé

It is not talking of love but living in love that is everything.

—A Yogi tea bag

I am brave, I am bruised
I am who I'm meant to be—this is me.

—Keala Settle,
The Greatest Showman ensemble

CONTENTS

INTRODUCTION

ONE DAY, I found myself, a forty-something-year-old single woman, urgently seeking, within the shelves of my local bookstore, solutions to what I saw as my lifelong problem: my inability to meet Mr. Right. I knew that my plight wasn't unique, but as I picked through book after book on relationships and dating, I didn't find anything that really spoke to me: the cookie-cutter how-to manuals; the sociological research about the cultural origins and present-day conundrums of the "spinster"; the bitch-and-moan dating escapades of a twenty-something who perceived the age of thirty as a line of demarcation between the chance to attain a lifelong relationship and never attaining one at all (not that I hadn't once also thought that way); and the colorfully packaged love advice of celebrities who had the privilege of fame, fortune, and makeup/hair artists (along with a very photogenic partner) on their side.

I searched high and low for a book written for and by someone who was like me, a regular woman who was working her ass (and heart) off to conquer challenging circumstances in the pursuit of love and life. I was looking for a book written by someone who'd gone through deeply personal struggles and who'd surmounted big obstacles. I was looking for empowerment, for an honest narrative with real life lessons that could teach me how to find success and happiness in love, pages that would show me, through someone's intimate journey, the way out of the single woman hole in which I'd spent decades residing in duck-and-cover mode. I needed someone to reveal how (and if) it was possible to find the love of my life, one arduous and courageous step at a time.

I was looking for my life partner, and when I didn't find him in the traditional manner in which my peers had found their significant others, when I thought I'd exhausted all options, I decided to write to him—and so this book was born.

I Just Haven't Met You Yet is my open love letter to my future life partner, chronicling my dating history, similar to yours or to someone you know. Each chapter begins with a letter, followed by narratives that portray my path to break free of destructive relationship patterns and overcome my fear of truly being seen by the world, sharing the transformative lessons I learned—from following the advice of friends, to figuring out how to listen to my gut, to knowing when might be the best (or worst) time to share my deep dark secret, to changing my troubled self-image, to finding what love truly is, and more— while confronting each hurdle along the way to meeting Mr. Right.

In the words of Vincent Van Gogh, "I am seeking, I am striving, I am in it with all my heart."

I Just Haven't Met You Yet

CHAPTER 1

I JUST HAVEN'T MET YOU YET

Dear Future Life Partner,

I thought I knew just how we'd meet.

We'd be classmates in college, or colleagues on the job. We'd meet in the office copy room, or on Match.com, or at an acquaintance's wedding at the table for guests without a "plus-one."

We'd find ourselves on a hike with the Appalachian Mountain Club some late spring morning, or on our bikes on the Minuteman Trail when we both stopped at Spy Pond to take in the view.

We'd never meet at a bar, because, disliking loudness coupled with drunkenness, we never go to bars.

We'd introduce ourselves to each other at the café we both went to every Sunday with our laptops, early, when I was writing my first book and you were answering what appeared from the expression on your face to be some very serious email. You were the guy with his gaze glued to the computer screen, until you took the chance to look up, at me.

You were the one at the adult education class who came over and asked, "Is this seat taken?"

It wasn't. I said, "It's yours."

I thought a mutual friend would set us up. We'd hit it off.

I thought we'd meet in the waiting room at the doctor's office when I tore a ligament in my wrist during a boot camp class at the gym and you broke your arm in a bicycle accident on Massachusetts Avenue.

I thought, when I flew out west, we'd be assigned the same row on the plane. I'd have the window seat, you the aisle. We'd say a brief "hello." At takeoff, I'd turn my back so you wouldn't see me becoming airsick, or hyperventilating from my flying phobia. You'd tap me on my shoulder and ask if I was all right.

I thought we'd meet on a crowded Boston subway, our bodies pressed together in the summer heat, the train stalling during rush hour, or on the commuter rail, like that couple profiled in the Boston Globe, *who talked day after day on their way to work, falling in love. Three years later, he proposed. She said yes.*

Yes, I believed we'd meet. Sure, I was being idealistic. I was conjuring up a future that relied upon stereotypical storybook circumstances, which do happen for some lucky singles—but such scenarios were my own magical thinking.

Love wouldn't happen according to my plans. So, when I found myself over a certain age, when my friends had found their mates, but my life wasn't the coupled way I'd once imagined it would be, I had to keep the faith. I had to stay optimistic. Though I sometimes felt discouraged, I wouldn't give up hope, because you were out there, too. The truth is, I'm a romantic, and I always thought that if I took the chance to put myself out there—really put myself out there—I'd find you.

This book is my journey from way back there to here with you: the ways I tried to meet you; the serious, the humorous, and the downright odd experiences I had in my attempt; the obstacles that held me back and that I worked so hard to overcome; the steps I took to conquer my fear of truly being seen by the world; and the many, many lessons I learned along the way.

This is my "tell all." This is my open letter to you, my future life partner.

Good Luck to Me:
My 1,000th Adventure in Online Dating

I WAS FORTY-ONE years old and I'd never been in love. I'd never had a long-term relationship, or any real romance at all.

When we met for our first date at Crema Café in Harvard Square that sunny August afternoon, I wore my leopard-print sleeveless dress. Shawn showed up in a suit. He introduced himself with his leathery tan cheeks, sunken slate eyes, gray-speckled sideburns, and a smile decorated with several silver crowns.

Shawn's online dating profile, including one photograph, painted a portrait of a smart, single thirty-eight-year-old lawyer, tall and fit with dirty blond hair and a love of hiking. In his bio, he stated that he valued long-term monogamous relationships and wanted to one day get married and have kids. I held the same priorities and goals.

As I sipped a glass of lemonade, I pondered whether a thirty-eight-year-old could resemble a man in his mid-fifties. I watched Shawn as he dipped a straw into his bottle of imported Coke, as he bragged that he was about to drink a soda "made with 100 percent cane sugar, not that fake corn syrup stuff."

Shawn briefly asked me where I worked and where I was raised, and then presented me with a lengthy summary of his interests and his family back-ground, mentioning that he was born and bred in Boston, that his parents were thirty-two when they gave birth to him, and that his father died "proud to have reached the age of eighty."

Revved up by his enthusiasm for his roots, Shawn grinned and leaned his head forward to suck on his Coke. His attention wandered to my chest.

I caught his eye. "How long ago did your father die?" I asked.

Shawn lost his straw inside the Coke bottle.

"Five years," he said, glancing around at the other customers at nearby tables, couples and coworkers and single people drinking cups of cappuccino and espresso and nibbling on pastries. He added, "I'm not as young as I seem."

"I know," I responded, feeling my jaw tighten. "How old are you?"

He looked at me briefly before his eyes shifted. "Fifty," he said as he tried to retrieve his straw with his fingertips.

"Really?" I asked. I was a writer, but I could do the math. He was fifty-three, fifteen years older than his profile had stated and more than a decade older than I was.

I studied his face. He blinked and fidgeted in his seat.

"Well, if age is a deal breaker—" he started. "You would've never agreed to meet me if I'd been honest about—"

"Age isn't a deal breaker," I interrupted, pushing the words across my tongue. "But lying is."

His bio had hooked me. I didn't like to be duped.

Shawn shrugged and said, "It's online dating."

I slid back my chair. I wondered if, at my age, this was all that was left of the pool of eligible bachelors. Why was I in my forties and still looking for the love of my life? Why was love taking so long to happen?

I blamed myself. I'd spent my teens and twenties abstaining from romance, despite wanting a boyfriend. During those years, I dreamed of sharing my life with a man at the same time I avoided facing an unresolved underlying issue: the sexual abuse I'd suffered as a girl. It wasn't until I was twenty-eight, debilitated by anxiety and depression, that I finally sought professional help. At twenty-nine, I was diagnosed with complex Post-Traumatic Stress Disorder (PTSD). While my friends were getting married and starting families, I spent my thirties in therapy three times a week, coming to terms with my past and working to overcome the obstacles that the abuse had placed on the development of my life.

I thought that if I worked hard enough I could catch up to my peers. I, too, could find my life partner.

I dated. I met men through online dating, speed dating, religious groups, hiking groups, adult education classes, meet-up groups, and singles cocktail hours. But I never felt a lasting connection with the potential partners who came my way. And the longer I went without finding "Mr. Right," the more I wondered if I'd missed my window for love. Still, I wasn't desperate enough to settle for just any available guy.

"I have to leave now," I told Shawn. I stood up. I'd been on many first dates, but I'd never walked out on one.

As I left I heard him say, "Well, good luck to you then."

Good luck? I thought, after this date, after so many wretched dates, I needed so much more than luck.

Walking home, through Johnson Gate and Harvard Yard, past the food trucks on the Plaza, crossing Oxford Street, I tried to reassure myself: I was on a different timetable than I might've wanted, but the well wasn't dry.

There were still plenty of fish in the sea.

On the Advice of Married Friends:
Getting Cultured

I WAS A single, thirty-nine-year-old whiskey virgin when I enrolled in "Whiskey: A World Tour," a two-week Friday night adult education class, to familiarize myself with the beverage for social situations and to meet eligible bachelors. I thought that becoming a liquor connoisseur would make me more cultured and therefore more interesting to a potential mate.

"But whiskey?" asked my therapist, Dr. Ross, cocking his head. After a decade of PTSD recovery work, my session topics were now gravitating more toward the common concerns of an average single woman rather than the details of my traumatic past.

Dr. Ross knew that I disliked drinking: I'd never enjoyed the way alcohol made my body relinquish its sense of guardedness or the way it made my brain feel fuzzy. But even more so, after an adverse withdrawal reaction to Klonopin, an anti-anxiety medication I took for a couple of years during the early stages of my recovery, I'd become almost entirely intolerant to alcohol. If I ingested half a glass of wine watered down with ice, my heart raced; if I drank half a glass of wine watered down with ice after 5 p.m., I developed insomnia.

So why on earth would I sign up for a whiskey tasting class?

My married friends said that whiskey was the new favorite among thirty- and forty-something males. I thought they ought to know; after all, they were successful in their search for a life partner and I wasn't. And I didn't want what I saw as my (distasteful) personal flaw (what adult didn't enjoy a good drink?) to get in the way of finding you.

At the time, I believed I had to offer myself up in an enticing way, hook a man like a fish. I didn't think I was enough of a "catch." I thought that, if I learned to enjoy whiskey, I might become more of the woman you were looking for. I didn't see myself as that woman already.

I'd originally registered for "Friday Night Wine Tasting: A French Wine Tour" instead of the whiskey class, because I thought it might attract a classy crowd; however, out of a waitlisted fifteen-person course, I was the only one who showed up. According to the instructor who looked like a maître d' in his pressed black suit, tie, and cuff links, everyone, except for me, canceled a couple of hours before start time.

I'd brought the two required wine glasses, but Mr. Maître d' informed me that I couldn't use them because they were for champagne. Wasn't a wine glass a wine glass? No, Mr. Maître d' insisted, it was not. He handed me one of his glasses, uncorked a bottle of Tripoz Cremant de Bourgogne Brut, and began to pour.

Watching the wine level rise in the glass, I proposed: "Maybe you want to reschedule for a date when more people can attend?" I was there to get educated, but I wanted to do it with others.

I tried to convince Mr. Maître d' to postpone by explaining that a glass of wine heavily watered down by ice would give me a buzz. If I drank more than that I'd experience a racing heart, I added. I'd panic from the sensation. I wouldn't be any fun.

"I just drove three hours to get here with two-hundred-fifty dollars' worth of wine in my trunk," Mr. Maître d' said. "I don't want to postpone. The point of a wine tasting is to taste, not swallow, though I do plan to swallow."

I couldn't think of a good enough reason or courteous way to excuse myself, so I stayed.

Mr. Maître d' launched into a demonstration of how to examine the color of wine in the glass, how to swish it. He stopped mid-sentence because, due to my left-handedness, my wine was sloshing rather than moving smoothly in the acceptable counter-clockwise motion: "Go clockwise instead," he ordered, "and you'll get the Coriolis effect."

I remembered the time my father suggested I demonstrate the Coriolis effect for my seventh-grade science fair project. I was out of ideas and had asked for his recommendation. I could do that, he said, or I could make beer. Beer seemed a common choice to make, but the Coriolis effect sounded original. My father showed me how to re-create the Coriolis effect in our bathroom sink; we watched the water's spiraling pattern as it went down the drain.

Mr. Maître d' demonstrated how to sniff wine, how to roll it over all of one's taste buds, and how to aspirate through the wine. He had orgasmic experience after orgasmic experience with bottle after bottle, while I racked my brain for a legitimate way to end it.

After an hour, anxious that there were still two hours of class remaining, I resorted to fibbing. "I'm feeling buzzed," I said. "I'm going to have to wrap this up now." I'd barely had three sips, though I did wonder if a person could become inebriated just by inhaling alcohol.

I didn't wait for a response.

En route to the subway, I passed a candlelit restaurant where couples were sitting beside the window, enjoying wine over a meal, looking at each other, in love. I knew their lives weren't perfect, but I envied them. I thought about my married friends who had no idea what it was like to still be single and on the verge of forty. Tears blurred my vision.

I was tired of being an observer standing on the sidelines of partnered life.

Determined, I purchased the two required Glencairn glasses for "Whiskey: A World Tour" and placed them in my purse, keeping the price tags attached in case I might want to return them.

That Friday night, I put on a skirt and top and my sexy black suede boots, careful to avoid my two rescue cats—Hannah, a crème calico, and Sam, an orange tabby—who wanted to rub up against my legs, so that I wouldn't show up to class with fur clinging to me.

"Go show them how it's done," said the big-bellied security guard who let me into the locked building, pointing toward the classroom. I peered inside and saw a long rectangular table dotted with paper plates that were piled with pretzels.

Sitting around the table were six burly male senior citizens who laughed with wheezy smokers' coughs; one dark-haired twenty-something woman who busied herself texting; two late-fifty-something women with what appeared to be hangovers; four thirty-something athletic men sporting Polo shirts and egos the size of a football field; and a woman my age, with an auburn-dyed bob and large breasts (which I wished my rather flat chest had) that she let dangle onto her copy of the typewritten list of twenty-seven whiskeys to be tasted in the ninety minutes of our first class meeting.

In the center of the table were two ice buckets, which I imagined were for either keeping the whiskey cool (I'd later learn people don't drink whiskey "cool") or vomiting. In truth, they were "dump buckets" for pouring one's excess liquor. Beside the buckets sat a red Target tote fashioning the motto, "Each bit counts."

Feeling like an imposter, I sat in an empty chair located beside the texting woman.

The instructor was a high school English teacher, a tall muscular man close to fifty with a rugged, unshaven face. Wearing jeans, a black T-shirt, and baseball cap, he stood confidently behind several rows of whiskey bottles, which were lined up like a set of bowling pins at the head of the table.

"My friend calls whiskey 'liquid asshole,'" he began, then explained that one ounce of whiskey is equivalent to one glass of wine. He recommended we consume no more than one-quarter ounce, "about the size of a pinky."

Whose pinky? I wondered. But I didn't voice my question, because I didn't want to appear ignorant. I was a college professor: I was supposed to be knowledgeable. Yet one of the consequences of socially isolating myself during my young adulthood was that I missed out on some basic life experiences. I felt ashamed of my lack of a certain worldly knowledge that I assumed everyone else around me had.

The instructor passed around the first whiskey bottle, the Buffalo Trace "White Dog," which he explained was made of 51 percent corn. I took a whiff: It smelled like nail polish remover. I didn't find the odor appealing. Was there something wrong with me? I didn't taste it.

Next was the Wild Turkey Russell's Reserve. "Notice," the instructor said, "how it smells of Old Spice, or mace."

I poured a splash in my glass and lifted it to my mouth, letting the whiskey wet my lips, which instantly began to burn. I decided I'd better not drink it. I put my glass down.

Two passing bottles later, I swallowed a tiny sip of the Four Roses Single Barrel, because the instructor called it "a beautiful, light, easy-drink." When it flowed down my throat it made me cough, hard. I felt like a teenager who'd just tried her first cigarette. I wanted to be like the other attendees who savored their tastings.

One of the senior men laughed at me: "You mean you haven't been a Scotch drinker for forty years?" He guffawed wheezily.

"We're gonna need more pretzels down here," called one of the thirty-something Polo shirt guys, pointing to the auburn-bob woman who'd been throwing back glasses one at a time. Now she was holding two at once. She squeezed her eyes shut, held her breath, and downed them. "We're gonna need more pretzels."

"Would anyone like the rest of my Pappy?" I asked, referring to the Pappy Van Winkle Buffalo Trace, which the instructor had said was a rare and very expensive whiskey as he passed it around the table alongside the George Stagg Bourbon. When I later told a writer friend, a woman who'd grown up in Kentucky, that I'd been acquainted with the Pappy Van Winkle Buffalo Trace, she suggested that either I was lying, or I'd been lied to; referred to as "liquid gold," the Pappy wasn't available, she claimed, not anywhere.

A Polo shirt guy turned to me, his eyes wide and hungry as if he were a boy in a candy store: "Me, me," he nodded.

The auburn-bob woman furrowed her brow. "You don't like it?"

"I'm just pacing myself," I said, feeling self-conscious. "I have low tolerance."

"I *have* tolerance," she said. "And I'm pacing myself." She threw back two more glasses, which I noticed contained more whiskey than the size of a pinky. She shook her head as if to recalibrate her mind. Then she leaned her head back over her chair with her mouth wide open and stayed that way. I worried about how she was going to get herself safely home.

The texting woman stopped texting and turned toward me. "My tongue feels funny," she whispered, chomping on it with her front teeth in a swift repetitive motion.

"Maybe you shouldn't drink anymore?" I suggested.

"Everybody have a pretzel," the instructor said. "Let's keep going."

———

That night, I remained the only sober one, dumping my whiskey "tastes" into the nearest dump bucket, which, halfway through, I imagined was a rather lethal concoction.

It's probably no surprise that I didn't return for the second meeting of "Whiskey: A World Tour." I'd learned well enough that I didn't like the beverage. More, I'd felt lonely there. I patted myself on the back for being open to the suggestions of my married friends, for trying something out of my norm, but I should never have taken their advice as gospel. I was my own woman, and I had to think like one.

Dr. Ross had been right to question my choice. I finally faced facts: Trying something out of my comfort zone was one thing, but I wasn't going to find my "match" by forcing myself to enjoy something I didn't, or by being anyone other than who I was.

Despite the letdown of my attempt, I remained optimistic that I'd find my "Mr. Right." I just had to try another avenue.

I just needed a more conducive setting, I thought: speed dating.

CHAPTER 2

LOOKING FOR MY SOUL/SOLE MATE

Dear Future Life Partner,

Do you think I was ridiculous, or brave, for trying that whiskey class?

I was determined. I thought my life would be more fulfilling if I could share it with a significant other, so I made a decision to remain open to any and all roads that might lead me to you.

Was being single such a problem? In and of itself, I didn't think so. I knew I could survive life as a single person—many people did (some even enjoyed it) and I'd already done so for my entire existence—but human beings are biologically and neurologically wired for companionship, and I was no different than the rest of the species.

I read many books on the plight of singles, including the confessional of a twenty-something fretting about not having a date lined up for a Friday night; a gimmicky "how-to, results guaranteed or your money back" anecdotal list of a book written by a relationship coach; and a research-based narrative that dispelled the myths of "spinsterhood" while explaining the negative connotation of such a status and its anthropological, sociological, and psychological underpinnings. While these books assured me I wasn't alone in my search for a life partner, none offered a viable solution.

I vowed to leave no stone unturned.

I enrolled in "Attracting Your Soul Mate," an adult education class with an instruction-manual approach to coupling. I thought that if I simply followed the correct steps, I'd find you. I'd stop what I was doing wrong and finally do it right.

"You must put yourself in receive mode," the teacher, a married-for-twenty-five-years wife, commanded. She lectured us—seven female attendees between the ages of thirty-four and fifty-nine—on the sexual and emotional aspects of her directive,

which I heard as plain old-fashioned submissiveness, a traditional role I wasn't will-
ing to play. She composed a list of activities that fell under "receive mode," enumer-
ating singles events and interest groups, routes I'd already tried many times over
without meeting someone I wanted to date. Were my standards too high?

I felt my chest tighten. I realized I was in the wrong place.

Real relationships weren't "order-up." While I could be open to meeting the right
person, actually encountering him—you—was an act of chance, which was ulti-
mately beyond my control.

I understood from experience that life doesn't always happen the way we desire or
plan, but I didn't want to passively leave love up to the universe.

How far had it gotten me?

First Impressions: Speed Dating

WHAT I LEARNED from speed dating is this: I can handle any man for six minutes.

When I arrived at the cocktail lounge in downtown Boston, I stood in line with several other women who were waiting to check in with Sue, our smiley brunette host who wore skin-tight, navy-blue jeans and handed out stick-on nametags.

The song "Freak Out" played from the loudspeakers.

"Where are the men?" one woman asked.

Sue giggled and rolled her eyes. "They're at the bar," she said. "Drinking heavily."

I turned and saw, in the dimly lit distance, the silhouettes of men sitting on a row of stools.

Don't get discouraged, I told myself, *not before the event even starts.*

I'd asked three of my single friends (two thirty-something women and a forty-something-year-old man) to come along to the speed dating event but they declined, citing a lack of money to pay the twenty-nine dollar entry fee, a lack of a desire to date, and (the man) "an inability to muster the enthusiasm" for a dating event.

So I went alone.

Beforehand, I researched how to succeed at speed dating. I read articles and watched YouTube videos, most of which were geared toward heterosexual men. Many warned prospective speed daters about becoming too tipsy before or during an event. Some discussed the art of the first impression, recommending asking your date questions that might spark a conversation rather than elicit a yes or no response. I thought that was good advice.

Sue explained that each woman was assigned a table and that, when the event began, the male attendees would rotate tables, taking six minutes to chat with each woman. When the six minutes were up, Sue would call out "time!" and the men would move on to the next table. She said the men might pretend not to hear her call "time!" but she promised she'd make sure they moved on.

I thought speed dating might prove more fruitful than online dating: Meeting someone in person, there was no guesswork about whether or not I felt an attraction, or whether or not the guy had lied about himself in his profile. I could appraise my potential boyfriend, and our connection (or lack thereof), three-dimensionally.

I went to the bar for a cranberry club soda and then took my place at my assigned Table #5. I looked at the numbered piece of paper Sue had handed me with my nametag, a slip she called "the scorecard." On the scorecard, I was to write the name of each man in the order I met him and check off whether or not I wanted to see him again. At the end of the night, Sue would collect the scorecards and, via email, send to any "mutual matches" each other's follow-up contact information. At the bottom of the scorecard was a tear-off section for any observations I might want to note along the way.

In order to make a good first impression as well as accurately evaluate the men I met, I knew I had to be completely in the moment, focused. My PTSD often prompted anxiety-induced distractions, but, as a writer, observation was my forte, and in dating it turned into a kind of "drishti," that point of mindful concentration I always heard about in yoga class.

As a girl growing up in an abusive home, I'd mastered the art of detail through hyper-vigilance, an enhanced state of sensory sensitivity and surveillance, a survival coping mechanism people in prolonged traumatic situations develop and reflexively employ to detect threats. I'd learned through therapy to tone down my hyper-vigilance into something less extreme and more useful to my present-day life: a keen sense of awareness.

In tandem, I was a good listener. I let the men I met talk and reveal themselves, their interests and values. While I listened, I asked myself, *do I like him? Am I attracted to him physically, emotionally, intellectually? Do I want to see him again?*

At the bottom of my scorecard, I wrote details about each man I met so that I could go back later on and deconstruct my perceptions, making sure I was thinking with my heart and not my past. Before my PTSD recovery, I was more concerned about whether or not my date liked *me*, versus my interest in him, and I blindly viewed men through the lens of my trauma, seeing a potential boyfriend as a type of perpetrator. In most ways I'd healed beyond that perspective, but sometimes I scrutinized my initial reaction: If I didn't like him, was that because I was seeing him through the veil of my history or was it because I simply wasn't interested in him? Sometimes the impetus was difficult to discern. I reminded myself I shouldn't be too picky as I could otherwise end up with no one—my mother always told me it was hard to find a good man. My father was the only man she'd ever dated.

As the event progressed, the randomness of speed dating reminded me of spin the bottle, the middle school game I only played until the moment the bottle stopped spinning, its nose pointing at me, or, if I'd spun, him, at which time I begged whichever boy I was supposed to French kiss in the closet to pretend we'd done it. Six minutes, next spin:

1. Mason: High school teacher. Lots of piercings but seems to have emotional depth.
2. Greg: Completely repelled by him physically and mentally. Talked and talked and talked and never came up for air: "I've been single for two years, medical equipment, import/export business, I hate being alone, what about you? I would like to be in a relationship with you, would you give me your email address?"
3. Lou: Really great energy. Co-owns family electrical systems business with his brother. Likes to hike and bike. The only thing I dislike: lack of eyebrows.

Was I being superficial? I challenged myself: Was I scanning for anything negative, for a reason why dating this or that guy wouldn't work out? Was the whole situation as absurd as it felt? I used my pen to cope with my nervousness:

4. Joel: Likes to "jump horses" and is "in a multifaceted support position" in which he writes reports of banks, webinar, has had fifteen years of Excel experience. Is this a job interview? Boring.

5. Antonio: Data scientist. Does "modeling and simulation." Something about a gun manufacturer? He was WEIRD and almost broke my hand while shaking it.

6. Nate: Is in the car repair business. Likes dragon boat racing.

7. Eddie: Does some kind of technology for a pharmaceutical company. Said something about a green card and "what're you looking for in a guy?"

8. Simon: Does hospital contracting. Likes golfing and scuba diving. Has the demeanor of a sixth grader.

9. Harris: Another data scientist. Asked me, "Have you done speed dating before? Is it better or worse than the last time?"

10. Will: When he sat down he gave me a thank you note with a printout of his name and email address and phone number. Said he likes pizza and hamburgers.

11. Shambho: He sneezed into his hand and then put out his hand to shake mine, saying, "Do you want to have a relationship with me?"

12. Doc: Stared at my chest while speaking. Told me he's named "Doc" not because he's a physician but because his last name has the word "doc" in it. When I asked what he does for a living he said he has an IQ of 176 but "is dumb as a crock" and is a lawyer. Has control issues: has to be the one to ask questions, not answer them. He only told me his profession after he asked me to guess his profession and I had no idea and had to ask him three times. Said, "Tell me about an experience you had that illustrates to me who you are as a person." Is this the Miss America pageant or a speed dating event?

13. Corey: Nice-looking, divorced, works in cancer research, likes classic movies, graduated from Yale. A little egotistical.

14. Las: Says that's short for "Douglas." Wants to write *Eat, Pray, Love*, the guy version. Not attracted to him.

15. Gary: Said he only had two beers before talking with me. Joked about having done shots at home before coming to the event.

16. Evan: Angry that I met him for an online date six years ago and didn't want to see him again and he couldn't figure out why. Scary angry.

I saw rage on Evan's face, which reminded me why I didn't want to see him after our first date six years earlier. As I took note of his clenched, white-knuckled hands, the back of my head tightened and my heart began to pound. Adrenaline stiffened my arms and legs. I felt myself detach from my emotions; I was dissociating, another trauma-based coping mechanism. I heard my voice outside myself, speaking in monotone, calmly asking Evan what he was doing these days. This was how I hid my fear. This was how I disarmed a man. And it worked. Evan's demeanor, to my relief, shifted from aggression to friendly pleasurableness as he told me he'd finished his degree in psychology at Harvard and was now planning to make money taking over his father's plastic clip badge–making business. Six minutes up—next:

17. Martin: Something about tech and artificial hip replacement (not sure if it's his own).
18. John: Picked his nose and shook my hand. Said, "I am at your disposal. I am a standard Indian product." (What?) Asked me how old I am, said he doesn't want anyone older than thirty-five. I said well I'm forty so I'm too old for you then. He said no, he'd like to give me a chance. Asked me how long I've been single. How long was my last relationship? I told him I don't answer such questions on first meeting. Said he's been divorced for two years and it's a truism that a person finds his match after one year.
19. Leo: From NY, went to U Michigan. Is a pilot for United Airlines, nice-looking. Talked a little fast. Not feeling head over heels but I'm open to seeing him again for a longer conversation.
20. Joe: Missing a few teeth, drunk, white hair. Told me he was retired and that I'm "too serious, you have to lighten up, you have to pinch my ass!" Repeated this over and over.

With Joe, I felt uncomfortable and irritated. I noted to myself how, in the past, I'd have felt afraid of such a man. "How much have you had to drink?" I asked.

"You need to loosen up," Joe howled again, slurring his words. "You need to pinch my ass!"

"I'm done," I said, dismissing him, sitting back in my chair. I surprised myself with my assertive response, but what surprised me more was that Joe didn't attempt to try again. Even though our six minutes weren't up, he went to the next table. I watched him sidle up to the woman there and lasciviously touch her shoulder and hair. The woman stiffened. For the rest of the evening, I watched Joe touch each woman at each table he visited. I felt disgusted, yet, in the moment, I didn't speak up. Instead, I questioned my reaction: *Am I making a big deal out of nothing?* Aside from some of the women's uneasy looks, no one protested. No one made a fuss or told him to stop.

Despite egging me on to pinch his ass, Joe had never tried to touch me. I heard a girl somewhere within myself ask, *Was I not pretty enough? Is that why?* No, I told that girl, I was pretty, that's why Joe had acted in a way he considered flirting. He didn't dare touch me because I'd put out a "don't mess with me" vibe. I'd taken Impact Model Mugging, a self-defense course, twice. I knew how to handle screwy drunk guys. While I didn't want to pinch Joe's ass, I could certainly kick his ass if necessary.

At the end of the evening, when I handed Sue my scorecard, I informed her of Joe's behavior, as well as my suspicion that he wasn't in the event's designated 37–47 age range. Sue assured me she'd pass along my comments to her boss.

Then I speed-walked to the subway station, dodging the rats on the stairs that led to the tracks—real rats, not men of a certain character.

———

Later that night, I received an email from the manager of the speed dating service, thanking me for reporting Joe, apologizing for the experience, and notifying me that she was banning Joe from future events. She encouraged me to return, and even dispensed a code for a fee waiver, but I didn't know if I'd go back, and not because of Joe, but because the men I met weren't, in my view, substantial boyfriend material. They'd tried to hook my interest with accolades and, at times, shock value. Such first impressions felt hollow.

It's hard enough for anyone over a certain age to find a decent date, but what I didn't see then was that my six-minute dates were reflecting a big barrier to my happiness in love: I was reenacting a dynamic that I'd had with my father. My father, a salesman and my first male role model, was all about the pitch. The aim was to hook someone into buying whatever it was you had to sell—material or immaterial.

I learned as a girl that I had to prove myself worthy.

When I was five, my father asked, "Are you pretty or are you ugly?"

I looked up at his freckled face, at his blue eyes and thick, fiery red hair. "Pretty?" I guessed, hoping.

My father gazed off in the distance, waiting a few seconds before responding, as if he were deeply considering the truth. Then he shook his head.

"Ugly?" I asked, wishing it weren't so.

My father shook his head again.

"No," he said. "You're pretty ugly."

Over the course of several minutes, my father asked the question numerous times. Sometimes he paused after the word "pretty," before he said the word "ugly," as if it were a trick. Then he broke into uncontrollable laughter.

At first, I was confused. Was "pretty ugly" good? The phrase contained the word "pretty." My father was laughing so I thought maybe it was good. But I felt something inside my chest fall, which told me it wasn't good. I was unlovable, and a joke.

My father's question became a regular inquiry for many months (it then grew more sporadic, until it faded out of style a couple years later). After a while, I learned to quickly answer "pretty ugly" so that he wouldn't have a chance to strike his punch line—I didn't want him to have the pleasure of the put-down, the win. But he worked around my defensive move. When I answered "pretty ugly," his voice turned kind and warm: "You're pretty," he countered, and I felt loved. But a moment later he asked the question again and his verdict changed to "pretty ugly."

For decades, whenever I looked in the mirror, I debated whether I was pretty or ugly.

My father taught me how I should expect men to view me. Speed dating brought my past to the table: My engagement with incompatible men, including some immature jerks, was a replay of my subconscious wish to somehow this time, this time, be good enough to make my father, and his interest in me, healthy, genuine, and enduring.

I was seeking real love the wrong way.

I still had work to do. I had to go back and unhook myself from certain life-defining moments, trappings of my past. Doing so was the key not only to unlocking the door to successful dating but to opening myself up to a real life on a variety of levels, and, in the process, to the possibility of a relationship with you.

CHAPTER 3

ON DISCLOSURE:
TO TELL OR NOT TO TELL

Dear Future Life Partner,

Let's be real: I've been scratching the surface, keeping things light, fearing you'll otherwise run for the hills. Yet there are deeper experiences I want to share, things that have shaped my life, that have brought me here.

I'm an open book, and yet I struggle with how to tell you my secrets. I don't want to over-share and possibly lose you in the process. Like you, like everyone, I have baggage. I'm not my past, but sometimes people have defined me by the things that have happened to me instead of seeing me for who I am. Can you relate?

Disclosure can be risky business. I don't have the power to control your, or any-one's, reaction, and I'm nervous about what that reaction will be. And yet, I think that withholding the truth is a greater risk. Doing so stymied my relationships for a long time. In my attempts to avoid revealing what I was afraid might result in judg-ment and rejection, I pushed away potential boyfriends. I came off as guarded even though I didn't want to be. My ability to engage and connect switched off. I discov-ered that trying to ignore or dodge or hide my past sabotaged my dates.

I've learned that it's best to just put the truth out there, to own it and then let the chips fall where they may. That said, I certainly don't go on a first date, or even the first few dates, and announce that I've lived through some trauma. However, when the past does arise in conversation, as it is eventually bound to do, I don't pretend that it doesn't exist.

I once believed my baggage made me less worthy, but then I realized my baggage is invaluable, because it gives me insight into how to handle problems as well as the ability to empathize with my partner's own struggles, increasing the capacity to bring us closer, to solidify our relationship. We all have baggage, but I believe it's not a weakness or a "red flag" unless we let it play out blindly and destructively; if we manage our issues in a self-aware way then baggage becomes an attractive strength.

When it comes to relationships—platonic or romantic—I'm all for transparency. I'd rather build something genuine, a bond based upon authenticity instead of falseness or shallowness. But when you meet someone—friend or partner—it's hard to know exactly when to tell that person about your history, when to share your greatest pain. And yet at some point it must happen if there's to be any real intimacy.

Does all this sound therapist-y? I'm not trying to be philosophical or highfalutin. What I'm trying to say is this: I don't want to only know the facts of you. I want to know the soul of you. And I want for you to know that of me.

But not everyone wants these things.

Once, I briefly dated a man who was kind, funny, attractive, and intelligent. We met on Match.com and our first date was the best first date of my life: We talked for two hours at a standing-room only bar—yes, a bar, and yet there I felt a rapport with this man as we discussed Seinfeld episodes, U2 songs, outdoor fitness activities, and our respective jobs. I thought we were compatible. I didn't expect that as the weeks progressed our relationship wouldn't, except physically and only in private as he wouldn't kiss me (except for a peck) or even hold my hand in public. When we made out, in my apartment, with the blinds down, I couldn't feel him, or even sense him, the person inside his body. While he hungrily shoved his tongue into the depths of my mouth, I considered whether my past was putting up a barrier, but my past wasn't what was at play.

He didn't want to be seen.

I assumed he'd reveal himself at some point; some wait a while before having sex, while others take the emotional aspect of a relationship more slowly.

On our second date, we were at an art museum observing a sculpture that we agreed looked like a person in a yoga pose (though it wasn't) when he mentioned he went to "Broga," yoga classes for men. I asked how long he'd been practicing. He said eight years, that he'd first tried it "during a difficult time."

"A difficult time?" I asked. He shook his head—he didn't want to explain right then and there, not in public he said. I didn't pressure him. He promised he'd tell me later.

Later, days and weeks came and went. Every time we were together I wondered about his "difficult time": Was it a bad breakup? He'd said he'd previously been in a serious relationship; for four years they'd lived together. Had his ex cheated on him? Was it depression? Alcoholism? Was that why he mentioned, "My drinking days are long behind me"? Did he have an STD? Had he battled cancer or lost a loved one to terminal illness? That might explain why he ran 5K and marathon fundraisers supporting cancer research, or why he shot me a stern "oh come on, what do you mean you never get the flu shot?" when I said I never get the flu shot.

Date after date unfolded the same: He talked to me over a meal, listing the superficial activities of his day, but when I asked what he thought or how he felt about this or that, or about the quality of his friendships, when I tried to find out what made him tick, what experiences had influenced him (the good, the bad, and the ugly), what he wanted in a relationship, what he wished for his present and future, what were his triumphs, what were his regrets, his dreams, when I shared such things about myself, when I showed my desire to know more about him, not just his itinerary, he changed the subject or made a joke or left the table for the men's room.

With him, I felt lonely. I was closer to acquaintances, to people I didn't even like. This wasn't a romance. This wasn't much more than a cordial exchange. But he was a nice guy. I thought there must be potential. I thought something would give way after he opened up.

A month in, I asked him to please tell me about his "difficult time." He hesitated, then finally disclosed what had happened: his eight-year-old niece had had leukemia when she was a baby. She was still alive and in fact had been healthy for a very long time. Everything was fine.

I expected him to add something further, some forbidden detail, but that was the entirety of his "difficult time," which he said was "a private matter," a secret that wasn't to be discussed with anyone. Not even his best friends or former lovers knew. I didn't understand why a common illness, and one that had ended well, and years ago, was so unmentionable. How did he—would he—cope with everyday problems, or anything worse?

I told him an emotional connection was important to me in a relationship; he said it was important to him, too, but described himself as "not very forthcoming in that aspect" (even his word choice was formal, distant). I asked if he might want to learn how to be. No. Then how was it important to him? I didn't understand. Then I realized we spoke a different language when it came to relationships. How might he react if I shared something unpleasant or challenging from my life? "I'd never tell you not to share something," he said. "But I likely won't have anything to say in return." He wasn't being insensitive, he was being honest; his words only confirmed my experience of him.

He said there was no good reason for talking about such matters, and if I expected to have such conversations, then he wasn't the right guy for me. I knew, with his stance, that we could never work through a conflict, an integral part of a partnership.

I didn't judge him—we're all built differently—or think I could change him. I took his words at face value. I said goodbye. He let me go. He wished me well.

I felt sad. His notion of knowing someone was vastly different from mine.

Same as one of my best friends, only I didn't find out until twenty years down the road, when she died of breast cancer, an illness none of her friends had known she'd had. After her death, I found out about a lot of things I'd never known, events that had occurred during the course of our friendship: She told me when her grandmother died, but not when her father passed or that her parents had divorced or that she was having a fifteen-year love affair with a much older married man, someone she'd said was "just a friend," someone whom, without my knowledge, she'd brought into my apartment when I was out of town, when I'd asked her to collect my mail and check in on the place. I'd find out these things after he informed me of her death, when he offhandedly and with a grin described the layout of my studio unit.

My friend had known almost everything about me, including my parents' divorce, my PTSD diagnosis and the sexual abuse of my childhood, along with the day-to-day goings on of my work-related and personal life. But after her death, I wasn't sure what we'd really shared. Had our friendship been anything more than a sham?

So here I am, putting my heart out there, looking for a man who'll do the same, understanding there are no guarantees, just knowing that that's who you are. And if that's not who you are, then you're not the one for me.

Take me or leave me: The truth is, I'm a deep person and I'm looking for a deep connection, mutual openness and vulnerability. That, to me, is what creates closeness. Trust and growth—that, to me, builds a relationship. I don't expect us to be serious all the time or even half the time; I crave levity, joy, and playfulness, too. Believe me, I want and need happy times. But the reality is, that's not all there is in life.

You see, on the road to meeting you, I came upon several detours that brought me back into my past, to the places where I'd left behind parts of myself I barely recognized, parts of my life I'd wanted to forget or had been too ashamed of or afraid to face. During such times, I felt utterly lost. I didn't know how or if I'd find my way.

While these detours seemed at first to take me away from my path, they were anything but circuitous. My past became a map that allowed me to make sense of where I was in my present (love) life. Looking closely at the intersections, stop signs, and dead ends, I saw my blind spots. In viewing the whole picture, I was able to recalibrate my inner compass. Only then could I position myself to go in the direction of the destination I wanted. Only then could I bring myself closer to you.

Only in removing the unspoken veil behind which a part of us hides can we truly let somebody in. And so that's what I'm about to do. Are you ready? Are you in? I'm going to show you where I've been.

My Deep Dark Secret

MY PARENTS DIVORCED when I was a college freshman.

"Your father is gone," my mother told me when I called from my dorm room a couple of weeks before Thanksgiving. "He left the house this morning."

"Dad took his things," added my brother, Russell, who'd moved back home to save money while working his first post-college job, "the lamp from the family room, the grandfather clock, the television set. He didn't even say goodbye, he just left."

I thought my father had left because I didn't love him enough. Or maybe he'd left because I loved him too much. Or, maybe he hadn't really ever loved me at all. Even if he'd wanted to, I thought, perhaps he just couldn't, or he'd tried, and it just wasn't possible, because of something about me, something deep within me.

And how could I blame him? I'd just left, too.

———

After the divorce, during my holiday breaks from college, and then graduate school, my father picked me up at the house to take me out for dinner and a movie. By then, Russell had moved to start a new job in a location too far to commute from our home, so it was just me going out with my father.

It felt like a date.

As my father's scheduled arrival time drew near, I began to have abdominal cramping and an intense urge to pee. I dashed back and forth from the living room window to the bathroom located down the hall every couple of minutes, then once a minute, then every thirty seconds (to try to quell my nervousness, I'd count the second hand clicking around the circumference of my watch), and so on, fearing my father would honk his horn while I had my pants down.

My mother watched me travel from the living room to the bathroom and back, perching herself on the mirrored armrests of our square brown chair, where I used to sit on my father's lap when I was a girl. Her face tensed and slackened with waves of anxiety. She told me she disliked when my father came anywhere near the house. She said she had nightmares about him trying to break in or suddenly appearing beside her in bed; she said he would never leave, even though he literally had.

She accepted the fact that while she was divorced from my father, I wasn't. I was his daughter, after all. Part of me wanted to spend time with him, while part of me didn't. I couldn't say why. I just kept hoping he'd be the kind of father that he wasn't.

My mother required that I greet him outside, at his car. I wasn't to let him come near the house, particularly the front door, which I was to double-bolt on my way out. I was to lock my mother inside: her orders.

The instant I saw him pull into the driveway, adrenaline jumpstarted my arms and legs and I ran to the door, opening and closing it as fast as I could so that he wouldn't catch a glimpse inside the house, so that I'd reach him before he got out of his vehicle. I was responsible for controlling my father and for keeping my mother safe.

I succeeded.

I slid into the passenger seat of the Lexus and shut the car door. My father flipped a switch and the locks went down. Beside me, the seatbelt was a dangling limb. In my head, I shifted into this second person:

You are here in this car. You're going out to dinner and a movie. You're twenty-two, twenty-three, twenty-four years old. You're not alone. I am right here with you.

Your father is behind the wheel, sitting beside you, looking at you, his palm leaning on the thick plastic knob of the gear stick, this thing between him and you. *What if his hand slips?* He leans over with a smile, saying *hello there*. He is happy to see you. See the way his eyes are glazed, streaming with jagged lines of blood that are scraggly on a milky background, streaking from the blue iris centers: centrifugation. His red hair is thinning, the strands now speckled with white, matching his unruly eyebrows.

Hi, Dad. Your eyes dodge his as if you're in traffic, trying to navigate through a collision course. Next to the gear stick is an empty coin dish. There's a black plastic cup holder beneath the radio and a coating of dust on the dashboard.

The heater exhales warm air on your cheeks. Beside the air vents are the radio speakers that vibrate with your father's favorite Phil Collins song, "In Too Deep." You want to close your eyes, but you keep them open.

Through the windshield, you view the brown-and-blue siding of the split-level ranch house and the stenciled flower-boxed windows that were once so beautiful. See the brief movement of a knit curtain, a hidden figure behind a dirtied glass pane. You look down, down, trace the ivy as it tangles around the rusted railing alongside the worn cement staircase, which winds in its descent like a petrified river, in steps, into the mouth of a driveway sea.

Dad takes your chin with his hand, turns it and lifts it toward his face. *I've missed you*, he says. A gold link bracelet dangles from his wrist. His eyes gaze upon you as he caresses your hair with one hand and pulls you in to him with the other. Your body resists slightly, politely. You don't want to hurt his feelings, you don't want to upset him, but you don't like this, you feel very uncomfortable. You can't say why. Above all, you can't say no.

You want him to understand intuitively, somehow, but he doesn't get it, or he does but he doesn't care; when your body holds back, the pads of his fingers pull harder, grip tighter around your jaw. Your sockets, your cheekbones, the back of your neck go chilled and nerveless. He holds you there. Tenderly, he put his lips to your face, not quite your cheek, but not directly on your mouth either, slowly, softly.

Is this really happening?

You remember how he used to kiss your mother hello—slow, soft, mouth open—in the front seat, when you were four and your brother was eight, in the railroad station parking lot where we waited in the heat for the train to come in, for Daddy to come home, for our family to become whole again.

Your mind becomes flooded so that all thoughts wash away. There is nothing but the smell of your father's foul, pungent odor. You hold your breath.

After he finishes he asks, *is everything okay?* You answer, *everything's fine, Dad.*

It's as if it happened to someone else. (Does he think you are someone else?) He lets you go and you let your breath go, though it goes shallow between your chest and your throat. Your pulse pounds in your temples.

You wonder if your mother saw it all through the curtained windows, if the neighbors did (you wonder if your father wanted them to). No one will ever say.

He *didn't do anything*, he says when you express discomfort; when you complain of his behavior he smirks, says *You sound like your mother*. He stuffs you with a wad of twenties. *How can you think that about me? It's all in your head—* his voice rises—*that never happened.*

Proof-poof: This is your father's mind trip.

Now I'm back in my body, fastening my seatbelt as my father shifts gears. He's taking me backward. We're leaving the driveway, the house, the world of my childhood.

He shifts gears again and we're en route to some other destination. I lean back in the cushioned leather passenger seat, a little disoriented, a little motion sick, a slight ache in my head, a sense of nausea rising from my stomach to my chest.

Years pass until someday down the road I'm no longer a passenger in this car. I'm in the driver's seat of my life with the steering wheel in my hands, the power to take myself to a better place.

I'll be the one who saves me.

Love Legacy

I SEE THE past as if through a rearview mirror in my mind: I catch sight of what's behind me, reflections of all that shaped my ideas about love, relationships, and my sense of myself, as a girl becoming a woman.

———

I had my first formal date when I was fourteen, with Ryan, a boy I thought resembled a young version of my father, only cuter and with glasses, who sat in the row next to me in English honors class. I was ecstatic when he asked me to our eighth-grade spring dance. He wore a suit, and I wore a pink dress with butterflies stitched into a lace bodice and matching one-inch heels. My father took pictures of us on the front lawn outside our home.

"Put your arm around her shoulder," my father ordered Ryan.

Ryan did as my father said.

"Yeah, like that," my father said, clicking the shutter.

In the picture, Ryan sports a macho man's grin, as if I'm a girl he's conquered, with my father's permission. I'm smiling, happy to have a date to the dance, a status I believed showed the world I was good enough, pretty enough: proof that I was on my way to becoming a successful woman with a successful life, someone who was obviously well-loved.

But behind my smile, in the secret crevices of my heart and mind and body, I was hiding a terrible silent sadness that I couldn't name. During the picture-taking, I stuffed down disparate states of feeling: titillation, confusion, and rage toward my father for commanding a boy to touch me while my mother, with her tightly curled blonde hair and sky-blue eyes, stood there watching.

When I got home from the dance, my mother asked if I'd enjoyed myself, if there were any slow songs.

Yes, I'd had a good time, and yes, there were a few slow songs.

"Did you feel him get hard?" she inquired.

The question made my heart race and my neck prickle. I felt alarmed, and dirty. I'd felt pride in being like the other girls who let their dates press their bodies against them (of course, the teacher chaperones monitored each couple's position, gently requesting a more vanilla stance if they saw things were getting "too hot"). That was the extent of it, though I didn't tell my mother this.

Did I feel him get hard? Was I supposed to? I wasn't sure.

"Yeah," I answered.

———

My father always said the truth was debatable. He said that if you cared enough about someone you could change your perception about what that person had said or done to you; you could change your belief to what that person wanted you to believe. To do so was an act of love, which resulted in a reward: acceptance, more love. I didn't realize this was a manipulative fallacy until I was in therapy in my thirties. Before then, I thought that if I disagreed with someone I must be wrong and the other person must be right, and I was afraid that if I expressed myself authentically everyone would think me unlikable for my crazy viewpoint.

When I was growing up, I believed my mother and I were close, but in truth that was a false perception. We weren't close, though my mother always said she was glad we were close because she and her mother never were and that was what she'd always wanted: a healthy mother-daughter relationship.

My mother always said, *I'm here for you.* She told me I could tell her anything. I was lucky: Other kids didn't have a supportive mother like I did. After I got home from school, my mother sat with me in the kitchen or on our deck and fed me a snack of apple slices and two cookies or a cupcake and asked me to share with her the goings-on of my day. She heard about my disappointments with friends or teachers and gave me advice.

I didn't want to admit, to my mother or to myself, that I didn't really feel that she was there for me. More often, our roles were reversed: I was there for her. She had a best friend, Nikki, who was my "aunt"—not my biological relative, but my mother's best friend from childhood—but in our house I was my mother's confidante. We often sat side-by-side in the recliner chair in the living room for what we called "sit and talk," our special time together. During "sit and talk," my mother asked me about my thoughts and worries and goals and dreams, but our discussions quickly turned into my listening to her talk about her problems with my father. She couldn't share such thoughts outside the home. She said if anyone knew what was going on, how bad things were between her and my father, they'd talk about us behind our backs. Nobody would like us anymore. We'd end up completely alone.

When I told her I felt sad, that I felt I no longer had a father, she said not to feel sorry for myself and that I was wrong, I still had my father. She corrected me: She said she was the one who no longer had her husband.

She told me she'd been happy in the marriage for the first ten years, but then something changed; she speculated that perhaps it was because Russell and I had grown older and she was evolving along with us but my father wasn't. He put on a "Mr. Nice Guy" act for everyone outside our house to see, she said, so nobody would ever believe how, in private, he was such a different person, sarcastic and demeaning, disrespectful of women's bodies and minds. He expected her to serve him; she couldn't be her own person. He was withholding money, and his feelings. She said they no longer had a relationship.

She spoke about her childhood, how her father often yelled and her mother often cried, how she felt unloved by her parents and her sisters, and how she frequently went to my Aunt Nikki's house down the street, the only place where my mother had felt a sense of nurturing and belonging. I was fortunate that we had such a close bond, she reminded me again, the kind she'd always wanted and needed but had never had with her own mother. She was glad, she said, that she could give that to me.

"Sometimes I forget," she stopped after a while, "that you're only fourteen."

———

I was raised in suburbia, Long Island, in the 1980s. My parents, Russell, and I lived in a split-level four-bedroom ranch house that my father refused to spend money on to repair even though it was rotting from the inside out, on a half-acre property with a properly mowed green lawn, a backyard of blooming flowers, maple and willow trees, and a basketball net in the driveway. My father worked in advertising sales in New York City; my mother was a housewife, writer, and, when I was entering middle school, a part-time copy editor for a book publisher. Russell and I went to public school; he played sports and I played the violin. My mother didn't let me wear makeup, except for clear or light pink lip gloss, beginning when I was twelve; when I was sixteen, I was allowed to add pastel eye shadow and blush. Eyeliner and mascara were not permitted; when I wore blue eyeliner at my college graduation, my mother frowned. She said I looked "hardened," my sweetness and innocence were gone. But I didn't think I'd changed, and I hardly wore any makeup at all. Still, with the back of my finger I rubbed off the eyeliner, as if somehow, in doing so, I could remove my mother's judgment of me, of my desire to be seen as a grown (read: sexual) woman.

When I was growing up, we belonged to a conservative synagogue where we attended services on high holidays and where the rabbi was ousted after a scandal broke in the newspaper. My mother told me he'd threatened his wife with a shotgun at their home and the police had been called. He was rumored to be having an affair with a congregant. My mother said she'd trusted him and felt betrayed. Later, our cantor, who always led us intently in song and prayer, would be quietly let go for allegedly molesting girls studying under his tutelage for their Bat Mitzvah. People talked, but only in hushed voices, whispering their gossip and disbelief behind closed doors, with many remaining loyal to our synagogue leaders. My impression, filtered through my mother's views, was that those who spoke out were shunned. My mother never asked me if the cantor had molested me, though I'd had Bat Mitzvah lessons with him weekly, sometimes twice weekly, for months. He never touched me inappropriately, though I always felt uncomfortable with the way he put his hand on my shoulder and stood so close behind me, his breath heavy on my neck, while I practiced reciting the haftorah. I never even knew of the allegations until years later, when I was in college and my father mentioned it in passing.

What happened in our community was a backdrop for what happened in our home. When I was twelve, Aunt Nikki (who'd introduced my mother to my father when they were fourteen) and her brother, my "Uncle" Darin, filmed and produced a movie as a surprise "gag" gift for my father for his fortieth birthday. In the movie, Uncle Darin played the role of a television reporter while Aunt Nikki acted out the character of my father, portraying him as an executive who barely performed his job, because all he was interested in doing was playing with a doll, a plastic little girl whose panties he loved to take a peek down. Whenever the doll was withheld from him, he'd demand to have her back, and he'd ultimately get his way. In the movie, he was called "a degenerate." At the end, his obsession with his girl doll caused him to lose his job, his home, and his wife.

Aunt Nikki and Uncle Darin were just kidding around. They knew my father liked dirty jokes, but they didn't know what was happening to me, though their attempt at parody tapped into the vibe of my more troubling actuality. When I finally confided in Aunt Nikki decades later, she recalled the video with sheer regret. "I didn't know you were being abused," she said. "But I'm not surprised." Through tears, she told me she wished she'd known at the time, and that if she had, she'd have done something. She'd have made sure I was protected.

As a family, my parents, brother, and I watched the video over and over again, sometimes multiple times a night, never growing tired of the story. Everyone laughed hysterically at the movie, especially my father. Back then, I didn't know what a degenerate was—all I knew was that everyone thought it was funny, and I was glad that we were with each other, and happy. When I became a teenager, and throughout my adolescence, I believed the story, with its humor, kept us together. My father couldn't *really* be a pervert; if he were, I thought, somebody would've done something to stop him. My mother would've made him leave the house or called the police. No one would be watching and laughing.

For decades, my mother held on to the video as a memento of a light-hearted occasion, keeping it as a fixture on top of the television set that she dusted every Saturday.

(As I share this, I wonder, in today's culture, in which experiences of sexual harassment and abuse are now openly discussed, if my father would've gotten away with the things he did in our house. Would anyone have thought such a "gag" movie funny? Would my mother have stayed with a man whose verbal threats she recorded in a miniature Mead notebook, words my brother and I would find hidden in her desk drawer after her death? Or would she have felt safe enough to tell someone, anyone, and get help? Would the abuse, and its accumulating damage, have been stopped? Would my life have turned out differently?)

———————

As a little girl, I felt loved by my mother, and safe, as we sat together on the black-and-white pinstriped couch in the living room in our house, next to the bright white globe lamp, with *Frog and Toad Are Friends* spread across our laps and my head leaning into the crook of her arm. This was a soothing backdrop to the unthinkable sinister reality that pervaded our home.

When I was four, five, and six years old, on Saturday mornings, after my mother went into the shower, I got into bed with my father. The yellow walls in my parents' room glowed with the morning sunlight as my father lifted up his sheets and I slid inside and closed my eyes as if I were going into a dream. I pretended it was a whole magical world down there. It was so warm with the heat of my father that it was a little hard to breathe at first, as if I were in the depths of the ocean, but I told myself I'd get used to it, I'd be like a fish.

When we heard my mother turn off the shower, my father said we had to stop. I could still stay in the bed, but we couldn't do what we were doing. Thinking my mother might catch us made my stomach flutter. I couldn't say why.

———————

Throughout my childhood, my mother was frequently focused on Russell, on his developmental issues. She was often caught up in his struggles, trying to get him out of his room where he would slam his door shut, trying to get him to socialize with other kids, trying to help him deal with the cruel ways boys at school would make fun of him on the bus or in the hallways where they knocked off his glasses and called him "four eyes" or "faggot." She held him close when he came home crying.

I loved my brother, but I was jealous of the special attention my mother gave him. I rarely allowed myself to feel or know the anger I held toward her for not also doting on me. Instead, I went to my father. He made me feel like a favorite.

My father liked to watch a lot of television on the couch in our finished basement. I could spend time with him if I lied down on the couch, beside him, so that's what I did. We lay together, my father with his arms around me. During commercial breaks, we did something my father called "making nice": We took turns touching and kissing the surfaces of each other's bodies.

Sometimes when we "made nice" we rolled around, hugging each other tight.

Sometimes my mother called to me from the living room upstairs where she was reading the *New York Times* or a novel she'd borrowed from the library. I heard her ask, "Trace, what're you doing down there?" and I looked at my father. He put his finger to his lips and smiled a silent "shhh" and held back a huge giggle as if it was really fun to deceive my mother, to keep what we were doing a secret. This was our game. We were partners in crime. We had a special bond. I called back to my mother with what I thought was a convincing "nothing!" or "we're just playing!" She didn't respond. I thought my answer had satisfied her, but after more time passed she called again, more sternly: "Tracy, come up here." Sometimes she left her newspaper or book and poked her head through the stairwell railing and said, "Trace, come here," in a serious voice that made me leave my father quickly.

When I reached the upstairs landing, my mother asked, "What're you doing down there?"

"Playing," I said. My eyes fell to the floor, averting hers. I knew I was in trouble. I'd been bad.

"Stop acting so wild," my mother said sharply. "Why don't you go to your room and read a book?"

It sounded like a punishment, but I was an avid reader, so I went to my room and I read a book and then I read another and another and if I ran out of books I read them again until I was so immersed in a fictional world that I became unaware of the reality around me. Reading felt like I was sleeping, only I was awake, disappearing into another life.

But I wanted to be with my father in the way a little girl does, and so I always returned to him, no matter the terms.

———

When I was eight, nine, and ten, at bedtime Russell walked by my room, where my father and I were under my covers, and went to his room, located next to mine, and slammed his door so hard it shook the walls. I thought he hated me. Looking back, I understand it was his manner of trying to intervene, to say *there's something wrong here* in the only way he, as a child, could.

Decades later, when I was in PTSD treatment and finally spoke to Russell about our upbringing, he told me he remembered how he used to walk by my room at bedtime. Over the phone, he recollected the scene as if it were a movie we'd all gone to see together as a family: "Dad would be under the covers with you and you'd be giggling. Sometimes the door was open and sometimes it was closed. I wondered what you were doing in there. I thought it was a little weird, and I was jealous of how much attention Dad gave you, so I'd go to my room and slam the door."

I didn't recall my bedroom door being closed. Throughout my childhood, my mother had a rule: My bedroom door always had to remain open, though it was okay for Russell to close his. I never asked why.

As a girl, I blocked out certain details of my experiences (a dissociative coping mechanism Dr. Ross would, years later, inform me was a natural response to the experience of overwhelming trauma), only to recover them piece by piece in my late twenties and early thirties. Russell's statements filled in some of the blanks of my truth puzzle.

"How long was Dad in there with me?" I asked.

"An hour or so," Russell said.

"An hour or so?" I questioned. My legs felt weak.

"It was for a long time," Russell said. "It went on most nights for a few years."

The sound of the door slam, the wall-vibration like a mini clap of thunder, or an earthquake, reverberated in the back of my mind.

"Where was Mom?" I asked.

"She was in the living room, reading a book or the newspaper," Russell said before he grew overwhelmed by my questions (how much could I expect he, or anyone, would be able to take of this terrible truth?) and changed the subject.

———

I remember how, one day when I was nine, Russell yelled at our father before punching his fist through the wall in our garage (Russell recollects it as not his fist but our father's). Later, he cornered me outside our house and said, "Why do you hang around him so much?"

I said, "Because he's fun." Because I needed to believe that was the reality. My father was my daddy, who taught me about my value and place in the universe, and how I was to be seen by men. I wanted the time we spent together to be the epitome of the innocent and affectionate core that motivated me to play with him. I didn't want that fantasy shattered. I didn't have the language to put it all into words then, but I was terrified of what the truth would mean for my family and for me, for who I was, for the person I was to become, for the kind of life I was to have. My father wasn't always abusive; sometimes I experienced him behaving in the way a father should with his daughter: protective, loving—like when I fell down and scraped my knee while playing kickball in the street with Russell and the neighborhood kids, and I started crying and he came running outside and carried me into the house; or when I was sick with the stomach flu and he sat beside my bed to keep me company and held back my hair when I vomited into the toilet; or when he took me to my Brownie troop's father-daughter square dance and bought me a fresh flower corsage from the florist, along with the "fake" flower version (made of plastic and fabric) sold at the dance hall, and do-si-do'd with me all night even though, according to my mother, he didn't like dancing; or how, before my first violin competition, he calmed my nerves and told me I could do it, and how proud he was when I did. Looking back, I sometimes wonder was all that pure, or was it grooming? Either way, as a girl, the idea that our bond embodied nothing but goodness was a lie I told myself in order to survive. I held fast to the belief that my better-behaving, loving father was the person my father really was, and that the other ways I experienced him were mere lapses, deviations in conduct and mindset that weren't his fault, but mine.

As I grew older, maturing, my feelings toward my father turned more complicated. Being around him was less "fun."

When I was about to begin sixth grade, my father cut off my mother's access to their bank account. Although she wasn't earning that much income copyediting, my mother opened her own checking account. When we went to purchase my school supplies, the store refused to accept her starter checks. My mother sent me to play with a rack of beach balls while she argued with the cashier and store manager; I was several feet away but I could still hear her angry, insistent, urgent, then semi-pleading voice; I could see her face turning dark pink.

Eventually, the discussion stopped, and my mother came to get me, her eyes wide and glassy. I'd spent a long time picking out the perfect binder with which to start sixth grade, but my mother said we had to leave it, along with the looseleaf paper, dividers, pencils, and pens. In the car, on the way home, she told me I'd have to ask my father to give her money so that she could buy the things I needed.

I remember the heat of shame on my cheeks and chest, as if my body was telling me I'd done something wrong by having needs. It was my fault that my mother was so upset.

I remember how I approached my father, my legs and stomach trembling as I sat next to him on his side of the bed he and my mother shared, beside the mahogany bureau where the checkbooks were located. As I stared at the scratched gold-colored handle of the closed drawer, my father bent forward, leaning his arms across his thighs and folding his hands between his knees. He said he'd dispense the funds, but I had to give him something in exchange.

I agreed.

Mid-sixth grade, when I was twelve, I told my mother I felt "uncomfortable" around my father. I don't recall her asking me why or in what way I felt uncomfortable, but as I stood in my bedroom doorway I heard her explaining to him in a half-whisper in the living room that my body was changing, I was becoming a woman, and I wasn't going to want to interact with him in the way I had when I was younger: "She doesn't like to play certain games anymore," I heard my mother tell him. She added that he needed to *understand.* He said he did. Then she told him she'd taken me to the store for my first bra, a triple-A cup. I couldn't believe she told him my size. I heard my father laugh. My mother murmured his name as if she were reprimanding him.

"I'm serious," she said. But then I heard her stifle a laugh, as if in commiseration.

"I know," my father replied, sounding as if he were trying to wipe a smile from his lips.

I was nothing but a joke.

Then I heard my father sigh, as if he were very depressed. He'd been sounding that way a lot lately. I felt sorry: I was hurting him by growing up, changing.

Later, we spooned on our basement couch in front of the television that was broadcasting *Who's the Boss?*, the episode where Tony, a widower, buys his twelve-year-old daughter Samantha her first bra. I hoped that maybe my father, by watching the show, would understand how I wanted him to interact with me, but instead he wrapped his arms around me and squeezed, with his hands placed just under my developing breasts. I knew he could feel my bra. I felt grossed out, embarrassed, and scared. But I didn't say anything. I thought there was something wrong with me for reacting so negatively, since my father seemed to think what he was doing was acceptable. I barely breathed so as to prevent him from further feeling the blossoming of my chest when I inhaled. On my exhale, I placed my fingers around my father's wrists, pressing his hands down toward my stomach, hoping he wouldn't notice what I was doing, but he did. He let his hands wander back to where he wanted them.

When I was thirteen, for many weeks my father frequently walked into whatever room I was in and sat beside me, his head hung low as if he were in mourning. He said nothing for many moments. Then he finally broke the silence by saying, "You know I love you, right?" as if it were a preface to something larger he withheld, to be shared only upon receipt of my answer, a kind of reassuring collateral. I answered "yes" and held my breath for what was to come, the announcement, but he never said anything else, he just sighed as if the news, the thing, was too terrible to even speak of, and patted my leg and left the room. I was confused because I'd answered "yes" so many times yet he kept asking, as if his need for the affirmation were insatiable. I felt graveness growing in the pit of my stomach, like a cancerous ivy wrapping around my gut, spreading silently, malignantly. I decided what it was, I knew it deep down: My father was dying. Perhaps what he had been trying to tell me was that it was because of me that all this was happening.

When I asked my mother if my father was dying, she frowned. She said nobody was dying. They'd started to see a marriage counselor, a family therapist.

"How old are you?" my parents' therapist asked from his maple-colored rocker stationed across from me in his one-room office, which was located in a finished basement at the rear of his family home.

His name was Dr. Tetley, like the brand of tea. He had white wild hair, a thin pink curve of a half-smile, and a translucent wart at the tip of his chin.

Dr. Tetley had counseled my parents for several weeks before he recommended they bring in Russell and me, "in order to help your father become more involved in the therapy," my mother explained to us privately the evening before we went: My father had been threatening to quit. He didn't see the point of going. He said he wasn't the one with the problem—someone else was the cause of their marriage troubles.

I sat on a dark brown sofa with my mother to my left, her palms lightly closed between her thighs. On the other side of my mother sat Russell, silent as a cumulonimbus drifting across a darkening sky.

My birthday had just passed. "Fourteen," I answered, rubbing the tips of my thumbs with my forefingers, focusing my gaze on the base of my nails, the half-moons of white, which was easier than looking anyone in the face.

"I see," Dr. Tetley said.

My father was sitting diagonal, to my right, in a large cushioned burgundy chair. From the corner of my eye, I saw his posture: at ease, amiable.

Nervousness numbed my legs and arms and ribs, surrounded my collarbones, wrapped around my neck. As the session continued, I went somewhere else in my head until Dr. Tetley jerked me out of my mental haze.

"One minute you want to be affectionate with your father," he said, his voice rising, "and the next you don't. How's he supposed to know?"

My father had mentioned examples, such as my sitting on his lap or letting him rub my head and play with my hair. Sometimes I liked it, wanted it, sometimes I didn't.

From the corner of my eye, I saw my father's posture: slumped, wounded.

My mind ran, searched for words, got lost in the glare of the light from the stained-glass lamp behind Dr. Tetley's back, got stuck on the end table, on the box of tissues waving its single white flag.

"He says you send mixed signals," Dr. Tetley pushed. "How's he supposed to know what's okay to do?"

I had no answer. I didn't know if Dr. Tetley would understand. I didn't understand. Anger rose in my throat. I swallowed it. Sadness pooled like warm blood in the cavity of my chest.

"I'm sorry," I said in my father's direction, but I couldn't look. "I'm sorry." I said nothing more. I had nothing else to give as consolation, reparation. I didn't mean to withhold myself from him. I was confused. I didn't understand.

"That's okay," my father said stoically, taking what words I had. From the corner of my eye, I saw him fold his hands in his lap: case closed, discussion over.

Bits and pieces of words wafted through the air after that, but I let it all go over my head like steam rising over a cup of stilled tea, vanishing, until my mother and father went at each other with furious tones: Then my body stiffened, my face turned warm and so did my limbs, except for my hands, which went ice cold. I had to go to the bathroom. I felt an intense pressure within my body. Thoughts flooded my mind. I was afraid of my father's anger; I was afraid of my mother's fear. I was afraid of the drive home. I was afraid we'd get into an accident. I was afraid I would die in a wreck.

I thought I saw Dr. Tetley look at me then, his spectacles catching a flash of light. I felt an urge to scream *please, please make it stop*, but my voice had left. I tried to say it with my eyes, until I realized Dr. Tetley wasn't looking at me after all—he was focusing over my shoulder, at the clock on the wall. He let time register in his mind, and then he looked away.

This was the end of the session. This was the end of all of the sessions. My father refused to return.

———

One night, after I went to bed, my mother walked across the lime-green carpet of my tiny room and sat on the edge of my pink flowered duvet-covered mattress.

"What're you going to do?" she began in a soft, somber voice, her body a silhouette. "Watch soap operas and live in a dream world for the rest of your life?"

My face grew hot.

My mother knew I'd become obsessed with watching *General Hospital* after school. But she didn't know that I secretly daydreamed of Chief of Police Robert Scorpio, along with his detective-wife Anna Devane, their younger officer-hunk Frisco Jones and his wife, Felicia. Every night, in order to fall asleep, I imagined they came to save me: Robert and Frisco broke down the door to the house and found me huddled in a corner of a barren room, stripped of my clothes. They saw that a man was hurting me. Robert and Anna arrested the man while Frisco and Felicia covered my naked body with a blanket and carried me to safety: *It's okay, it's okay*, they repeated, comforting me. They cared for me. They took me back to their home on the outskirts of Port Charles, their city, and sat with me for hours, holding my hand while I cried, asking me to tell them what had happened. I was too upset to speak, too ashamed. I was in shock and on the verge of a breakdown. Once Robert and Anna were done booking the man at the police station, they arrived at Frisco and Felicia's place. Anna and Felicia were like protective mothers, making me feel safe, encouraging me to tell them what had happened. They said they'd sit with me until I was ready to talk: *He can't hurt you anymore. You're with us now.*

Finally, I told them: The man had touched me. The man had raped me. I didn't know how I'd be able to go on living. I didn't know how I could survive such a truth. *It's alright*, they consoled me, *you're going to be okay now, you're safe, we're here.*

I desperately needed someone to trust, someone to take charge, to help me feel safe, though I couldn't say why. I didn't have the knowledge or vocabulary to really understand or speak of what was happening to me. Sure, I'd watched the after-school specials on stranger danger, and both my parents had sat my brother and me down to watch the *Diff'rent Strokes* molestation episode, but that molester wasn't the child's father. I understood good touch versus bad touch. But I didn't understand family systems theory or sadism or denial or incest. I felt afraid all the time, but I couldn't say why. I just wanted someone to tell me I was going to be okay. I wanted someone to say that my fear that my life was over before it had even begun was unfounded. I wanted someone to show me there was still hope.

My mother lowered her lips to my cheek and kissed me goodnight. "You need to learn to be self-sufficient," she said. "Don't look for a man to take care of you. That's what I did. You have to be able to take care of yourself."

To my mother, marriage was a prison with a husband as warden. It was better to be alone. I had to learn to live without a man, without my father. In truth, I had to learn to live without my mother, too. I had to be able to take care of myself, and before I was capable.

Although I yearned to be rescued by Robert, Anna, Frisco, and Felicia, I knew they were fictional characters. The actual people I had in my life to take care of me were my parents. And I didn't want them to get divorced, because I thought they'd die without each other, and I thought I'd die without my parents.

Every night when I went to bed, I enveloped myself within my dream about Robert, Anna, Frisco, and Felicia so that I could sleep, so that I could escape the fact that there wasn't anyone real who was going to save me.

This is something I'm embarrassed to share.

As a teenager, I felt like my father's girlfriend, a role I detested, loathed, and feared, yet at the same time such a dynamic made me feel important and cared for, an object of love. I thought such a romantic association was a sign of perversion: mine, not my father's. I blamed myself for wrong thinking, not my father for wrongdoing. I thought that if I tried hard enough, perhaps I could change my perception about the way things were.

Like any straight teenaged girl, I fantasized about making out with boys my age, but never went further than first base in my thoughts. When I masturbated, I entertained no fantasy at all. I closed my bedroom door and went into a kind of trance state. I focused on spreading a blanket of blackness throughout my mind's eye. Sometimes an image of a man intruded, and I fought it, him, tried to blot him out with more blackness; other times I succumbed to an uncontrollable forbidden arousal. I touched myself, but it was more like I was abusing myself instead of pleasuring myself (and not in the colloquial "abusing myself" way people kid about masturbation). Whether or not I climaxed, I'd be rough and insistent on my body until my skin was raw or bled. Whenever my mother saw my door closed, she knocked and opened it (I was breaking the open-door rule), sometimes without waiting, consequently interrupting me, asking me, with her cheeks stiffening, what I was doing, as if I were a sexual deviant, though she said at least I wasn't getting it from a boy. I was mortified. My mother never normalized my sexual feelings or taught me what healthy sex was. Years later, she'd tell me my father had called her a prude.

Perhaps these details verge on "too much information" for my life partner or anyone to hear about, but if I were to leave them out I'd be withholding part of my story for no other reason but my shame, and such shame belongs not with me but with my father and mother, yet that shame is still, after all these years, hard to shake. If I were a man writing this book, the topic of teenage masturbation would not be glossed over or omitted, but would be expected, a given. Truth: Girls are sexual beings, just like their male counterparts, one of the many reasons why sexual abuse is so harmful, especially during the crucial years of sexual development, yet (and perhaps as a result of needing to deny the fact) many people deem incest too "taboo" to honestly and openly—as opposed to sensationally and ignorantly—talk about.

———

On the bureau in my parents' bedroom, my mother kept an eight-by-ten black-and-white photograph of my father's high school yearbook picture. One day, she gave it to me to keep on my night table. She didn't want his face in their bedroom anymore. I felt torn with it in mine.

My mother told me that my father's face "lit up" when I walked into the room. Her voice was tinged with resentment.

———

In my mid-teens, I was my father's prized possession. He took pleasure in picking me up from my shift as a candy striper at the local hospital. He pulled the top down on his convertible and turned up the music. When we stopped at a light, he put his hand across the backrest of my seat and looked over at the car in the lane beside us, as if to say to the driver, *look at my girlfriend.*

I believed I was hideous in the eyes of everyone who saw me, and that I was becoming that way to my father, too.

"You were really cute," my father often told me, "when you were five."

I thought I was becoming too old. I obsessed about my inability to stop aging. With each passing day, I was becoming less and less special.

———————

The idea of becoming an adult woman filled me with sickening anxiety. All the other girls at school seemed to want to grow up as quickly as they could, but I wanted to stop time.

I knew my thinking wasn't normal. When, during "sit and talk," I told my mother about my concern, she suggested I write to Abigail Wood, the column editor of the "Relating" department at *Seventeen* magazine, for advice. I had a subscription to the magazine and thought my mother's idea was sound. Within a couple of weeks, Abigail Wood sent a letter in response. When it arrived in the mail, I took the envelope to my bedroom, where I sat next to my stuffed animals and tore it open, relieved to finally have a solution in my hands:

Thank you for writing to Seventeen. We're glad you felt comfortable enough to confide in us.

We assure you that what you're feeling is perfectly normal. In fact, you'd be surprised to know how many readers write to us with the same concerns that you have. There is really nothing that anyone can say that will make you just stop worrying. You write that you know you can't control or change time. Since you realize that, then why don't you focus your energy and thoughts on making the present the best possible for yourself? Concentrate on looking forward rather than always looking behind you.

We've enclosed articles that may be of some interest to you. We also encour-age you to talk about what you're feeling with people who can offer you support and sound advice—like good friends and your family.

I considered that perhaps Abigail Wood hadn't really read my letter and had sent a boilerplate response, but she'd signed it in blue ink, so I thought it must be personal.

The enclosed articles addressed issues of time management and applying to college. While I planned to go to college, to me leaving home meant going out into a world I believed would be the same as the one in which I was growing up, only on a much larger scale, a place ruled by domination and my expected sub-mission and powerlessness.

Despair enveloped me, and I tossed the correspondence aside. While I thought Abigail Wood's advice was good, she didn't understand: I wasn't "per-fectly normal," and now I didn't believe my problem could be fixed.

I learned to ignore the truth, and to bury it deep. But then something would happen, jarring me out of my daze, making my heart pound and the adrenaline pump through my limbs.

One day, during our family vacation, I was swimming in the pool at the resort where we were staying. In the distance, I could see my mother sitting supine, her legs and feet stretched out on a lounge chair like a paper weight, her head and torso hidden behind the *New York Times*, the tips of her fingers hold-ing it open across her upper body as if the publication were a shield from the life that went on around her.

I dreaded climbing out of the water, the way my bathing suit clung to my skin, the way my father always stared.

Standing at the pool's edge, my father planted his eyes on the V-shape of my body where my legs met my hips, where I felt the water drip. I saw his irises turn hard, and hungry.

I felt like prey.

Silently, quickly, I walked past him but not so fast as to show my discomfort or fear: to reveal a reaction, an emotion, would mean to be caught, and subsequently consumed.

I breathed shallowly to contain my reaction, though I felt my heart pounding past my collarbones, up my throat to my jaw, as if I were trying to escape from my body through the exit of my mouth.

Finally, I reached the lounge chair next to my mother, grabbed my towel from where I'd left it, and wrapped it tightly around my waist.

"Dad's staring at me in my bathing suit," I said, keeping my voice out of my father's range, barely above a whisper, though I felt alarm licking at my throat like the uncontrollable flames of a fire. I swallowed to try to extinguish it.

I heard a sigh and the newspaper rustle before the top edge parted, unveiling my mother's face, her eyes on the page, her pupils moving across the words, taking in the news.

"Cover yourself up then," she said, sounding annoyed, or afraid—I couldn't tell which—by my father or by me, by my body.

After that, I wore a long baggy shirt over my swimsuit, or simply avoided swimming. I thought my body was abnormal and disgusting. I wore only loose-fitting or bulky clothing, never anything that defined my shape. I covered up my body, my heart, my mind, my memories, my experiences, layer after layer of, year after year, until I became so numb to reality that I no longer recognized my life, or myself.

When I was an English major in college, dabbling in communication courses, my television production professor asked me to stand up in class as a model example of the type of clothes one should never wear on camera: She pointed out how my large sweater made my body appear as a blob, how my sweatpants and turtleneck masked my contours. I felt strangely disoriented by the truth—wearing such clothes had become my unconscious habit. My unattractive body was plainly obvious to the other students. My professor pointed to another girl named Tracy, a sorority girl I envied for her beauty and popularity. She wore skin-tight jeans and a tank top, the perfect outfit, my professor said, in which to be seen.

I had my first real kiss when I was twenty. When I say "real" I mean "appropriate," as in, of my own volition, with a peer.

I was a college sophomore, at a Hillel Hanukah party, standing in a stranger's kitchen with Bernie, a junior computer science major at a university about thirty miles from mine, in the city. I'd met Bernie at a previous Hillel gathering. He was mild-mannered, short and thin with a large shiny nose. I liked him, because he seemed nice, nonthreatening. I wanted to kiss him, date him. I wasn't all that physically attracted to him, but when he leaned his face into mine, I placed my mouth on his. His lips felt like tiny balloons: rubbery, puffy. Later, we made out in the dark corner of a hallway. I let him put his hands up my sweater, but when he tried to touch me under my bra, skin to skin, I stopped his fingers with my own: *no*. He didn't push further.

At another Hillel party, he invited me up to his dorm room. I thought he wanted to show me what it looked like or just wanted to kiss in private. But when I saw his room, which was so small it only fit a tiny dresser and a bed on stilts, I didn't want to move past the doorway. Feeling fear rise in my stomach, I suggested we go back to the party. He didn't object.

Bernie was a safe choice for a boyfriend: He didn't pressure me to see him or to have sex. That was easy, because we lived a forty-five-minute drive apart and neither of us had a car. We talked on the phone once a week, but we rarely spent time together. Still, I could say I had a boyfriend, like other college women: I had proof of my normalcy; I wasn't the "freak" I thought I was.

Despite the warnings my mother gave me about men—"they only want one thing," she always said, pursing her lips—she ultimately wanted me to get married, and to a Jewish man. Dating Jewish wasn't just her stated preference for me, but my requirement, a stamp of approval of my innate goodness as a person. I wasn't to date outside our family's religious faith. My heritage was important to me, but I thought the dating rule was unfair and closed-minded, yet I wasn't brave enough to consider defying my mother.

When I was home for spring break, my mother asked if I liked Bernie. I said I thought he was nice, but I wasn't head-over-heels for him. She said it was hard to find a nice Jewish man, and if Bernie was nice (we already knew he was Jewish), then I should try my best to make sure things worked out.

I mulled over in my mind how my mother had married my father, a Jewish man, and how badly that had turned out. But I thought she knew best. I let her rules and beliefs make most of my decisions, even if those decisions went against my heart. I thought I had to obey her wishes in order to remain loved by her, and to be lovable to the world.

Yet, shortly after my conversation with my mother, I did break up with Bernie. I knew, in truth, that we didn't have a relationship, and I'd grown tired of pretending that we did. Merely saying I had a boyfriend was no longer enough for me. What was the point of dating someone I wasn't really dating and didn't really like? I wanted to *really* date someone. I wanted to have a real connection. I wanted to feel attractive and attracted to a good man. I wanted to truly be with him, despite my unacknowledged abuse-driven fears around sex.

Bernie tried to convince me that we did have a real relationship. He said, for example, that he'd sent me Valentine's Day chocolates (so had my father). But I'd had enough of the façade.

Still, I wondered, what if I'd passed up my one opportunity for a life partner? What if Bernie was my only shot? What if my mother was right? She'd married the first and only boy she'd ever dated. Of course, she'd gone to college when most women went for their "MRS" degree and were considered doomed to spinsterhood if they weren't engaged by graduation. Times were different. But what if the truth was that there wasn't anyone else out there for me?

———

I thought that maybe a real dating life was conceivable during my senior year, a couple of weeks before my twenty-second birthday, when I received an email from someone with the username "PigsFly."

"PigsFly" told me that he was a secret admirer who'd seen me around campus. I was excited. I asked questions, trying to guess his identity. He responded evasively or in flirtatious riddles. He told me he'd reveal himself on my birthday.

I hoped "PigsFly" was Jordan, a tall and handsome guy I liked in my English literature class, but I didn't know how Jordan would know when my birthday was, unless he'd asked my friends. But my friends told me they hadn't talked to Jordan. They couldn't guess who "PigsFly" was, but, like me, they couldn't wait to find out.

When my father called the following week, I mentioned the emails I'd received from "PigsFly." He was intrigued. He asked if I had any ideas about who this "PigsFly" was. I mentioned Jordan but said that otherwise I really had no clue.

I longed for my birthday to arrive, for the day I might acquire a true boyfriend.

On my birthday, I waited for "PigsFly" to reveal himself. I waited all day, but I heard nothing. I began to feel impatient. Then, the phone rang. It was my father. He laughed and laughed and laughed.

He was "PigsFly." I'd fallen for him.

It was a joke, my father claimed, but I didn't think it was funny. I thought what he'd done was horrible and sad. But I didn't tell my father what I thought, because I didn't want to face my humiliation. I told myself it was my own fault: I'd dared to think that I could be a normal young woman.

When would I have a real boyfriend? When pigs fly.

This was my love legacy.

CHAPTER 4

CROSS MY HEART

Dear Future Life Partner,

I know, that was a lot to take in. But I see you're still here. You haven't yet run for the hills.

I've come a long way since those awful days.

My upbringing was built upon a self-destructive belief system that I wouldn't learn to dismantle, or even become aware of, until my thirties. Until then, my dating life was like one of those "no turn" traffic signs, my heart surrounded by an impenetrable red circle with a canceling line crossing diagonally through its center.

Confession: I spent years expecting abandonment, particularly from men. The reality is, I abandoned myself. For decades, I kept my spirit buried underneath protective layers of denial until I was in a place and time when I felt safe enough to begin to resurrect myself, piece by piece. I had to first find the courage to stand by myself before I could expect anyone else to stand by me.

When I look back at my younger self, I barely recognize the person I showed to the world: As an adolescent and young adult, I was passive and meek. Outwardly, I took things in stride. I never exhibited a strong reaction to anything. I never cried in front of anyone or grew visibly angry. Instead, I got quiet, in the way I did the summer I was seventeen and working as a cashier at CVS when, during my second week on the job, I was held up at gunpoint while manning the register. My father had driven me to the store that morning for the start of my shift. Coincidentally, he'd instructed me on how to behave if I were ever robbed: Keep your hands down and your voice compliant, he said. Pretend nothing bad is happening. Do whatever the robber says. Give him everything.

And that's what I did.

I saw the weapon wedged between his tight blue jeans and pale flesh, how his fingers curled around the wood-colored handle of the gun. I focused on the aisles of merchandise lined behind him, rows of packaged black combs, foil-wrapped chocolates, and One A Day multivitamins. I listened to Lenny Kravitz singing from somewhere above: So many tears I've cried / So much pain inside / But baby it ain't over til it's over. . . . *I saw another customer approach the checkout counter. Her fake red nails tapped the top of each bottle of shampoo in her plastic shopper's basket.*

The robber said, Hurry. Give me the large bills, the ones you hide, *he pointed,* underneath your drawer.

My manager was in the back room, located behind a mirrored wall that overlooked the store. The mirrored wall served as a security decoy; in reality, it was a one-way window from which the manager could see everything, including the robber and me. But she didn't see, because she was focusing her attention on counting change: quarters, nickels, and pennies in their proper slots.

I was new at using the register, and not very skilled—my previous summer employment had consisted of alphabetizing books at my local library, a job more aligned with my introverted nature—but I somehow managed to reflexively hit the no-sale key to open the register drawer. I removed the wads of wrinkled bills, singles, fives, and tens and twenties, which I handed to the robber. Looking at the vacant drawer, I felt a void spread inside me.

So many years we've tried

to keep our love alive

'Cause baby it ain't over til it's over . . . (over, over)

I was so calm, so acquiescent that even the customer with the shampoo bottles waiting behind the robber didn't realize what was going on. She just kept unloading her shampoo bottles onto the counter. When the robber turned to leave he said to her, "Have a nice day, ma'am," *and she lifted her eyes for the first time and responded,* "Thank you, you too," *as if he were a perfectly nice man.*

When I paged my manager by picking up the phone and pressing the intercom button for the back room, privately informing her of what had just transpired, she became hysterical, quitting her post and running down the aisles yelling at people to get out, throwing the remaining customers out of the store and locking the doors. After the police arrived, I called my mother to tell her that I was ready to come home, hours earlier than scheduled, because I'd been held up at gunpoint and the store was now closed for the rest of the day. My mother said I must not have been in any real danger, because if I had been she'd have felt it. She told me that a mother has a sixth sense about her child's well-being.

She sent my father to pick me up.

When he arrived, he shook his head and said, "None of this should ever have happened." He wasn't referring to the robbery, however, but to his and my mother's impending separation.

A week later, I identified the robber in a lineup after he'd been caught holding up another store. He went to jail. The money ($250) was never recovered. In the end, my manager fired me for "giving away" store funds.

A few weeks after the incident, my mother urged me to see Dr. Tetley to talk about the holdup. She said I wasn't "acting right," I was "quieter than usual" and she was worried about me. I didn't think I'd been behaving any differently, but the way my mother had noticed my need for help made me feel taken care of, which was comforting, so I agreed to go.

During the session, Dr. Tetley didn't seem interested in the robbery. He kept steering the topic toward my relationship with my father, telling me to extricate myself from a dynamic he called "a triangle" between my parents and me.

He said, "Don't let your father make you his little wife."

I knew my mother had seen Dr. Tetley for individual sessions to help her cope with my father after the couples counseling had stopped, so I thought perhaps his statement came from what he'd gleaned from her. But I didn't like the fact that he wasn't hearing me. He didn't seem to understand that I didn't have the power to control my father, just as I didn't have the power to control the robber. Yet he talked about it as if it were my responsibility.

––––––––––

"Did the surgeon remove part of your brain when he took off part of your breast?" I heard my father say with bite.

I was standing in my bedroom doorway, listening to the silverware sparring with food on the dinner plates in the kitchen. I imagined my father cutting his meat with the jagged edge of his knife. There was silence. I imagined in the silence that my mother, who was recently hospitalized for the removal of a borderline-malignant lump in her breast, was dishing more peas onto her plate, letting them tumble in circular patterns, poking their middles with the points of her fork.

Pots and pans crashed on the linoleum kitchen floor. The sound lodged itself in my ribs. Taking a few steps to the hallway closet, beside Russell's vacant bedroom (he was away at college), I retrieved a thick towel and then tiptoed, barefoot, toward the bathroom, located halfway between my bedroom and the kitchen. I counted each step, feeling my skin brushing against the bark-colored carpet, until I reached the cool tiles of the bathroom floor: safe.

I closed the bathroom door, pressing the lock securely in place, then undressed quickly, piling my clothes on the countertop by the sink. I stepped into the shower and turned on the faucet to drown out the sounds of arguing.

The steady stream of hot water filled my ears, pelted my back and flowed over my body, warming my shoulders and chest. Shutting my eyes tightly, I prayed the arguing would be over when I turned off the water, but when I did things were worse.

When I told my friend Leila that I was upset that my parents were having marital problems, when I told her I didn't know how I could bear further turmoil, she said, "I'm not worried about you." She said there were people she worried about, but I was not one of them. I was the type of person who could handle anything. Of course, I hadn't told her about the worst of it. I hadn't told my own self.

I could handle anything and everything. I numbed myself out in order to do so.

Early on in my PTSD recovery, Dr. Ross explained dissociation, how a person can "go someplace else" in his or her mind to escape an experience that is threatening or otherwise unbearable. That was how I pushed away what was happening and even blocked out some of what occurred, until I was in a physically and emotionally safe enough place, as an adult, to fully grapple with the traumatic details. Dissociation allowed me to grow up as an overachieving student in high school and college. I

became an adult whom clinicians in the trauma field labeled "high functioning":
I was a woman with an advanced degree, an apartment, a full-time job, and a
relatively stable, though socially isolated, life. Other survivors coped by developing
severe Dissociative Identity Disorder (DID) or addictions, or led a life of crime and
prostitution, or became homeless. Some were hospitalized for psychotic breaks. Early
in my recovery, when I participated in a trauma education and coping skills group,
out of ten adult childhood sexual abuse survivors in the room, I was one of only two
who engaged in conversation. The others sat around the table coloring with crayons
for self-soothing. Sure, I had some issues, but I managed.

I was lucky.

In my thirties, although I felt unlucky in love, I was on a journey to untangle my
heart from my damaging past. The men I met, the dating experiences I'd try to
navigate, the relationships I'd attempt to have, would show me the way. I just didn't
know it yet.

Teenage Love

I HAVE REGRETS. But I've come to have compassion for my younger self, and to understand the pain that kept me from finding Mr. Right for so many years.

As a teenager, I didn't think of myself as "normal," but in many ways I was. I had a crush on Matty, a reserved boy with round wire glasses who played clarinet in the school band and sat behind me in ninth grade honors earth science class. His assigned hallway locker was next to mine. I thought that meant it was fate that we date.

Matty and I had a similar kind of social shyness so I thought we'd make a good couple, like Kevin and Winnie on *The Wonder Years*. But whenever I attempted to flirt with Matty, a bully named Josh ruined everything, approaching from behind so that I didn't see him coming, lifting my skirt and running his fingers through my hair. He wrapped his arms around my chest and groped my body and whispered dirty things in my ear and shouted, "You're so sexy!"

Time and time again, he molested me in front of Matty, who stood there as if he were paralyzed, until he managed to regain his muscle power enough to take his books from his locker and give me a side-glancing look of apology before he scurried away to class. I was convinced that in his eyes, in every boy's eyes, I was sullied girlfriend material. Every time Josh touched me I became more and more unattractive.

Josh's harassment had actually begun a couple of years earlier, in seventh grade. Once, he lifted my skirt while I was walking up the stairs and I turned and pushed him down the flight, astonished by my own strength. But that only fueled his desire. He came back with greater force, again and again. Nothing stopped him, until I reported him to my social studies teacher in eleventh grade. My teacher, a man in his fifties, asked if I could think of any way that I'd elicited such attention. Had I brought on such behavior? I knew I hadn't, but I questioned my conviction, simultaneously feeling anger and betrayal surge through my body in response to the reaction of a trusted adult in whom I'd confided. I quickly smoothed my feelings away, afraid of uncorking the deeper well underneath. Had I caused such abuse to happen? I said no, but I debated whether or not my answer was correct. I gauged the veracity of my answer based not upon my own perception but upon the judgment of those in authority.

Ultimately, the school dean gave Josh a warning: If he ever bothered me again, he'd be suspended from the school athletic team on which he played. To my relief, he finally relented.

———

At my Sweet Sixteen party, everyone knew I wanted Matty to ask me to dance, but he hid in a crowd of boys, avoiding me.

In a video that my cousin's boyfriend took of the party, I appear frozen in my first off-the-shoulder dress, an emerald green taffeta, as I stand in front of a pink and white sheet cake, candles lit. The DJ runs through what we're going to do next—on the count of three, I'm going to lean over and blow out the candles and then everyone will sing happy birthday to me.

I'm staring at the light of the candles, as if part of me has melted into the glowing wax.

"Tracy, are you awake?" the DJ asks amusingly.

His voice jolts me out of the haze of dissociation. I look up and smile and say "yes." But the truth is I'm barely present.

After the candle blowing is done, and the guests have sung, the DJ announces that my first dance will be with the guy I've known the longest. He tells me to go get him. I think that he's referring to my brother, but when I start in Russell's direction, the DJ interrupts: "Think *carefully*," he says. "The guy you've known the *longest*."

I'm confused. What boy is the DJ talking about? My friend Ethan shouts out "Matty!" and giggles ripple through the room. The DJ quips: Never in all his years of Sweet Sixteens has a girl messed up which guy she's supposed to pick for her first dance. I stand in the center of the dance floor feeling chagrined. My mind spins.

I see my mother mouth, "Your father."

My father bashfully pokes his face through the crowd of my peers. I feel frightened by the rage that suddenly springs inside my chest—for the fact that I have to dance with my father instead of a boy my age, for the fact that my father's body language shows he's hurt by my not thinking he's the guy I'm supposed to pick, and for the fact that everyone sees I'm guilty of an unforgivable mistake. I hold my breath. I swallow my anger and shame. I try to be a normal and good girl.

I want to be like other girls who partake in the father-daughter dances of special life milestones, so I do what everyone expects: I reach out my hand. I invite my father to come to me. He walks over, puts his arms around me, and pulls me close. I hate the touch of his warm shirt against my chest and collarbones, but I want to be fine with it, I want to like it, so I pretend I do. We begin to slow dance and I feel everyone in the room ease. The DJ plays "Happy, Happy Birthday Baby," by The Tune Weavers. As I dance with my father, I disappear into a space within my mind where I can fast-forward to a moment in the future, to a plot I can create, control.

Later that night, the DJ plays "When I See You Smile," one of my favorite songs by Bad English, and I walk up to Matty, who's standing off to the side of the dance floor, and I ask him to dance. I hear a tinge of yearning, an aggrieved insistence, in my voice. Matty doesn't protest. He barely opens his mouth as he says "okay." He follows me onto the dance floor like a somnambulist.

On video, I'm beaming. Matty shows a self-conscious smile.

I was feeling happy for getting what I wanted. But I was also thinking that maybe it didn't truly count as dancing with Matty, because I didn't believe he did it of his own volition. I thought I'd forced him, similar to but different than the way my father had forced me to do things with him, things that, deep down, I really didn't want to do.

———————

Throughout high school, Matty remained rather aloof around me, though he did invite me to a party at his house, which I attended. I don't recall much about the party, except that Matty had just started dating a girl named Rochelle. I wondered why Matty was so enamored by Rochelle. What was so great about her? What was so lacking in me?

Eventually, I did move on: I developed a crush on Matty's best friend Matt, whose locker was located on the other side of mine.

While Matty sat behind me in honors earth science class, Matt sat in front of me, since our teacher had assigned seats alphabetically. Like Matty, Matt also sported intelligence and wire-rimmed glasses, but unlike Matty, Matt had smooth olive skin and matching eyes. He frequently turned around to whis-per-sing songs to me, with lyrics he'd make up in his head, spontaneously expressing a thought or sentiment regarding me or our class or his general mood. Many times he almost got me in trouble for laughing out loud at his songs in the middle of lessons on tectonic plates and the laws of the universe.

I never told Matt that I liked him, but during our senior year I was secretly hopeful that he might confess romantic feelings for me when he sent me a friendly valentine as part of our National Honor Society chapter fundraiser. I sent him one, too. But neither of us revealed any romantic feelings for one another. Did he like me? Did he know I liked him? I'd never find out.

We graduated and didn't keep in touch. Years later, in my mid-twenties, I tried to find Matty and Matt online. I thought that maybe I could have a sec-ond chance with one of them. I wanted to salvage something I'd wished for but had never had in high school: a boyfriend. I didn't want to accept my loss: the void of my teen dating life. I didn't want to see the underbelly of it, the destruc-tive impetus: abuse. I wasn't yet ready to accept the truth. I thought I could bypass it if I could only prove—by finding a way to develop the relationships I'd missed out on—that my upbringing hadn't irrevocably harmed me or altered the course of my life.

Searching online, I found Matt's email address. I messaged him, and he responded. He was completing a master's degree in biochemistry. He'd just pre-sented a paper at a conference on cancer research. He now preferred to be called "Matthew." He sounded so much more mature than he had been in high school. I thought maybe we might soon find a way to meet up, but then he stopped writing back.

Several years later, with the invention of Facebook, we reconnected again. He was Facebook "friends" with one of my Facebook "friends," and so I clicked on the "friend request" button. He accepted. He was living in Florida, happily married. He and his wife had had a baby girl.

I felt left behind, selfish and wistful. Life had gone on without me, and there was nothing I could do to change it.

———

In high school, Matty and Matt were "safe" boys—unlike Mark, who sat next to me in economics class. Mark was blond and broad and big-boned like a football player. He played softball. He was a joker and a jock. I felt out of his league.

"Gee, did the bell ring yet?" asked our economics teacher, Mr. Jones, with biting sarcasm and a slur he'd acquired from a stroke that had permanently affected his speech.

Mr. Jones had a helmet head of black hair, a big nose, swollen cheeks, alabaster skin, and an ornery mood. His face turned beet red when he yelled at students who didn't know the correct answers to his questions. Mark, who sat next to me, told jokes under his breath and imitated Mr. Jones's voice and mannerisms. Something let loose in me and I began doing the same. Whenever Mr. Jones yelled, Mark and I rolled our eyes at each other and choked on giggles. I'd thought Mr. Jones was a scary man but Mark helped me to see him as almost harmless.

Mark tapped into the innate playful and affectionate part of me that, by my teen years, I'd learned to suppress. Sitting next to Mark, I felt safe enough to be mischievous. I felt like one of the cool kids, no longer the nerdy girl the popular crowd made fun of for my high grades and frizzy hair and lack of fashionable clothes. Mark made me feel like I was one of the attractive school cheerleaders, which both enthralled me and made me nervous.

One day, Mark drove me, and my violin, home from school. When he pulled into my driveway, he asked me out. I said yes.

That Saturday night, when he came to pick me up, he knocked on our front door and my father invited him in. As Mark walked upstairs, my father followed, appearing slightly sheepish, as if he were out of place, a second wheel to my new prospective boyfriend. I pushed away a sense of guilt I felt bubbling up and shifted my attention to my mother who stood at the edge of the landing. I was waiting and hoping for her approval. She greeted Mark by putting out her hand. Mark politely shook her hand and said, "Hi Mrs. Strauss, pleased to meet you," as he peered over her shoulder at our diamond-shaped hallway mirror.

My mother smiled. "I hear you play ball?"

Mark's attention was caught in the mirror, where his face flickered like a self-interested, or simply self-conscious, teenaged boy. "What kind?" Mark responded, keeping his gaze on his reflection.

My mother shot me a look, as if she were trying to keep herself from bursting out laughing. Later, in private, she would comment that while Mark seemed nice he didn't seem very smart. She thought I could find a better boy to date. I liked Mark, and I felt disappointed by my mother's perspective at the same time I reflexively took on her judgment as my guide.

I shuttled Mark out of the house quickly.

We went to the local bowling alley where Mark paid for my shoes and our lane. He came up beside me while I waited for the ball return, his hands teasing their way around my waist and hips. My body was ticklish, and I responded with anxious laughter.

Mark kept throwing curve balls that landed in the gutter. I won the first game without really trying. Mark asked if I wanted to play another round. I said yes. His hands became more insistent and my body tensed. I stopped responding with laughter. Mark's demeanor became more serious, quiet. I won the second game and he said it was time to go. I thought we were going to dinner after bowling, but Mark drove me straight home, in silence. I thought I'd done something wrong. I felt embarrassed. I wondered if he thought I was a prude.

When we arrived at my house, Mark parked his car and walked me up to the front door. I thought he might kiss me. I felt excited as he leaned in: He'd be my first. Then I felt his breath and I suddenly felt afraid. I turned my face so that his lips landed on my cheek.

We hugged. I could tell by the way Mark hung his head that he was disappointed. I was disappointed too—with myself.

He left me on the doorstep and drove away.

———————

Mark came down with mono shortly after our date, so it was probably a blessing that I didn't kiss him, but barring that, the seventeen-year-old part of me who wanted to be a normal girl wished we had locked lips. Other girls my age were having sex with boys, and I hadn't even kissed one.

In the months following our date, Mark rarely talked to me. I didn't know if that was because of me or because of the mono. He was very sick and out of school for weeks. It never occurred to me that he kept himself at an arm's distance out of respect, because I'd signaled I didn't want him to be any closer.

That spring, Justin, a friend and classmate, asked me to our senior prom. I said yes, because I didn't think any other boy would ask me, and I knew Justin wouldn't try to touch me, as he was too polite, and I wasn't physically attracted to him, so I wouldn't be pressured or have to deal with any of the associated scary feelings I had around intimacy. These weren't the best of (or even admirable) reasons to say yes to a date, but I didn't want to miss out on going to my prom. I felt guilty when Justin sang Mariah Carey's "I'll Be There" to me on the dance floor, because I realized then that he had romantic feelings for me and that, by accepting his invitation to the prom, I'd led him on. At the end of the night, when the limo dropped me off at the house, he offered to walk me to the door. I told him no. He stood there in the street, closed his eyes and puckered his lips. I told him I'd had a great time, and then, feeling sorry, I awkwardly, rudely, left him on his own.

———————

A couple years later, I ran into Mark at a college party. He was friends with one of my floormates, a woman who'd invited him to visit. Mark behaved like a drunk party animal, though I didn't know if he was actually inebriated or if that was just how he let loose. I told my college friends about our date in high school, and they all agreed it was a good thing I hadn't let him kiss me. Deep down, though, I was trying to convince myself I'd done the right thing. I was trying to assuage my regret.

The summer after college graduation, I was living in New York City, working at Lifetime Television as a fellow with the International Radio and Television Society Foundation, when Mark called and asked me to meet him for dinner. Remembering my mother's words, I felt hesitant, but I agreed. Over Italian food, Mark put on what I saw as a show, sounding to me as if he'd rehearsed his lines. I perceived him as delivering a salesman's pitch. He told me he'd messed up in high school, but he was a changed person. He wanted me to give him another chance.

I said no.

I liked Mark's attention. But something about him reminded me of my father's personality. My mother had always said the only thing a man wanted in a woman was her body. Sex wasn't a mutual act of pleasure and closeness; sex was about a man's physical gratification and domination. Were all men like my father? Only, I thought, the ones who were attracted to me.

Looking back, I sometimes think, what would've been so bad about giving Mark a second chance? But I never would've done it. I didn't trust him. More, I didn't trust my own viewpoint. I lived within the realm of my mother's beliefs. I told myself I could find someone better, which at the time was an excuse to avoid examining my fears about being in a relationship, of knowing, and being truly known to, someone.

———

A little over a decade later, Mark "friended" me on Facebook. I was genuinely happy to hear from him and accepted his request. We were in our mid-thirties. I'd been through a lot of therapy. The way I'd been in my teens and twenties seemed so foreign to my sensibilities. Mark had married that floormate of mine, and they'd had a couple of kids together. He was working in real estate: He built houses and managed properties and had a sales license. "Life is good," he wrote through Facebook messenger. "No complaints here. How about you? What's your story?"

I told him I was living in Boston and working as a college professor.

He said he wasn't surprised. "You were always smart," he said. He mentioned our dinner in New York City. He said he wanted to clear the air:

I'd felt that I "crapped" in the well and I wanted to make amends for that by taking you to dinner, and at the very least apologize if I had hurt you in any way. I never intended to do so. I realize that this message comes to you many years after the fact, but all I can do is say I'm sorry. I hope that we can build a friendship of good memories from high school days and keep each other informed on our lives.

The dinner hadn't been a rehearsed pitch. He'd meant every word. Now, I didn't know what he was apologizing for. I thought I was the one who'd messed up by not taking his words at face value—I had experienced him through the lens of my then undiagnosed PTSD. I felt I was the one who'd messed up by not kissing him on our high school date. Mark responded:

I heard that you really liked me and I basically treated you like crap. I realized that over the years and I just wanted to right that wrong. [Growing up,] I had my own issues, my parents were selling the family home due to divorce and I became a bastard to deal with. The economics teacher had a stroke and a slur, but the class was boring and he was always late. Truth be told, I switched my schedule [the next year] so that I could be in the same Government class as you, because you always set me up to crack jokes between us.

I found it comical that Mark thought I'd set him up. I'd thought he'd been the one setting *me* up. He told me he was never much of an athlete, contrary to my impression of him, and he had his own share of problems with fitting in. I hadn't known that he was the target of teasing by some of the girls in the popular crowd. In turn, I told him what had been going on for me during those years, what was happening in my home. I told him about the sexual abuse. I told him that was why I'd dodged his kiss. I'd spent a long time wondering whether that was the reason he'd subsequently dropped me.

I'd grown confident enough within myself to know implicitly that I really could trust Mark. In turn, he responded in a kind manner that moved me:

Whatever you had going on, I never saw a glimpse of it. You hid it well. As a guy, we see things very black and white, especially when it comes to girls. I thought we had an enjoyable time [on our date]. At the end of the night, I recall walking you up to your front door and going to kiss you goodnight. Not sure if I was going for the lips or cheek, but either way, you backed off. NOW I UNDERSTAND WHY. (WOW!) Needless to say, we didn't go out again, but stayed friends. (I figured you were not interested in me that way.) I did like you. I was a bit dopey and broke. I spent my money on the bowling that night. I had no money left. BTW, if I didn't like you, I would not have tried to give you a kiss. As for dodging a kiss, knowing me, that's probably one of the reasons we didn't [go out] again. Especially, since I was a horny teen guy, a girl dodges a kiss from me, it's over in that regard.

I've realized so many things that I should have figured out when I was younger. I also realized that I was kind of a jerk in HS too. I thought I was hot stuff. I had a car, I could go places, etc. But I also realized that being a teenage guy I was a horny bastard and if I didn't hook up, forget her. Looking back, you pushing away was probably the one thing that saved our friendship. Otherwise, our "relationship" would have lasted about as long as wearing a pair of socks does, short-lived.

High school drama, glad it's over. By the way, I know you will find Mr. Right. Just remember, not all guys are Josh or Mark for that matter. There are good guys out there. You just have to be open to the opportunities when they present themselves. Trust in the process, Tracy. You'll find your bliss. I know you will.

Mark's honesty and faith in me truly touched me. When I was in high school, I didn't understand innocent overtures like Mark's. I saw sexual encounters, even flirting, as sinister, not innocent—at least those involving me (those involving anyone else I believed were "normal" and "good"). What a gift, I thought, to have Mark tell me these things now, two decades later. What a blessing to have him in my life.

Mark and I continued to stay in touch. His friendship helped to normalize my sense of my male peers, to untangle the visceral leftovers of past experiences from the reality of my current encounters. When I went on dates, Mark offered advice and reassurance, and, from time to time, to alleviate my nervousness, he dispensed the humor I remembered from high school: "Gee, did the bell ring yet?" And my nerves would transform into laughter.

As I began to publish essays about having PTSD, about overcoming the abuse of my childhood, Mark gathered more of the details of my story. He expressed his shock and sadness and told me he saw my strength. He offered the pure love of a friend.

To this day he continues to tell me that if he'd known what was happening to me when we were kids, he'd have helped me.

I believe him.

How to Fall in Love Without Really Trying

I ONCE BELIEVED age stacked the dating odds against me. But, as they say, with age comes wisdom. With wisdom comes perspective. And putting past relationship failures in perspective can give us the confidence to move forward. Examining where we've been shows us how far we've actually come.

———

I almost fell in love when I was twenty-three.

His name was Daniel Oxford and we met while we were both working as graduate fellows at the university writing center. I was pursuing my MFA in screenwriting and Daniel was completing his master's in public relations. Daniel liked to chat about *Seinfeld* episodes in between tutoring clients. In some ways I thought he resembled Jerry Seinfeld: He was average height, thin and clean-cut with short brown hair.

Okay, so that describes millions of men in America.

Daniel had smarts, and charisma, and he chose me (*me*, I thought, *out of any other woman he could've picked*) as the subject for his "Writing for Publications" class profile assignment:

She's afraid to leave her apartment in the morning. She fears going out at night. She even suspects that someone tapped her phone.

Tracy Strauss, the sweet and thoughtful graduate student who sits across the table from me at a Brookline Au Bon Pain, reacts to a bizarre situation like any normal and sane person might; I'd worry too, I think to myself, if I had become entangled with a man who now sits in jail for allegedly conspiring to commit murder. But the woman whose bright blue eyes, wavy blonde hair, and rosy face remind me of a cherub, has her own special weapon with which she transcends even the most challenging of circumstances.

I wasn't sure I liked his comparison of me to a cherub, but I was smitten with most of the rest of his writing. When we first met, I thought of Daniel as just a colleague, then as a friend. I don't recall when exactly I began to think of him as more than that, but the day he referred to his long-distance girlfriend Marcia in the "ex" category, I looked across the room at my best friend Lauren, another graduate fellow, and she looked back at me with a grin. She knew: I wanted Daniel to be my boyfriend.

Although Daniel didn't know it, seeing him on an almost daily basis gave me a reason to stay in graduate school. In my first semester, I was contemplating dropping out, because I dreaded going to my required "Acting for Non-Actors" class where my professor, an actor from a popular television series, sexually harassed me. A large domineering man, he frequently positioned himself as my partner for improvisation exercises. Cornering me, he'd start a dialogue about dating; when I froze and my mind went blank or I didn't respond, he became angry, scolding and shaming me into engaging with him. He talked about my hair and my body. *You're beautiful.* He touched my face and shoulders and eyed my chest. *You don't look a day over sixteen.* During a class exercise on motivation, he sat me down in a chair and offered me twenty dollars if I'd perform sexual favors. I went numb.

I told myself I was being too sensitive. This was an acting class. My professor was just "acting."

To my dismay, our paths began to cross outside of class. One day, at the crowded university dining hall, my professor showed up at the table where I was sitting by myself. He asked if the empty seat was taken. Before I could answer, he placed his tray across from me and sat down. I stopped eating. He lectured me on ways I could improve my performance in his class.

I had nightmares that he cornered me in a hallway and assaulted me.

The sexual harassment evoked visceral feelings from the past I'd buried, a truth from which I'd do anything to flee. I told my program director that I was considering leaving school, because I didn't think I could continue to go to my acting class.

"He's been sexually harassing female students for years," my program director said with exasperation at the situation. He encouraged me to continue my studies and arranged for me to switch into a different section of the course.

My new professor was displeased, since several other female students had also transferred in, overloading his class. On my first day in the black box studio, he asked me to stay after, to talk privately. I felt nervous. He wanted to know why I'd left the other class section. I didn't want to tell him the truth, so I responded vaguely that I didn't like the other professor's teaching style. He asked me to explain further, to be more explicit, but I simply repeated myself. His voice was stern, which I interpreted to be laden with judgment. I withheld the fact that my former professor had harassed me, because I worried my new professor would think I'd made a big deal over nothing and would therefore dislike me and make me his target, too.

———

Although I wanted a boyfriend, I was afraid of being the object of a man's interest. I thought there was something wrong with me because I seemed to attract the wrong kind of men: the stalker type. Two of my classmates, Jack and Ray, were examples. They asked me out and wouldn't take my "no" for an answer. One day, Ray somehow figured out my class schedule and showed up at the university T stop on my way home at 10 p.m. to "just say hi." I told him he was scaring me. *Please stop.* He finally did. Jack persisted, until I told him I was interested in somebody else.

Not all of the men I encountered were aggressive or incognizant of boundaries. Daniel certainly wasn't. And neither was Cullen, a thirty-two-year-old film production major with whom my new acting professor paired me to perform a scene from Woody Allen's *Stardust Memories*. I was to play a sex-crazed fan and Cullen, a gay man I thought resembled my celebrity crush, Richard Dean Anderson, was to play Woody Allen's role. The assignment was contrary to both our personalities. Instead of rehearsing, we talked about how much we dreaded the prospect of performing the scene. I shared with Cullen the truth of why I'd switched into the class, and Cullen told me that what happened wasn't my fault. We became good friends. Eventually, we memorized our lines, and we gave a performance our professor called "very convincing."

Later, Cullen asked if I'd critique one of his script drafts for a film he wanted to produce, and he read one of my screenplays, telling me he thought it was well written, but he wondered why there weren't any sex scenes. "The entire script lacks any hint of sex," he said. His tone was absent of judgment; he was simply stating his observation. "Sex is a part of life," he said. "Is there a reason why you don't write about it?" I brushed the issue aside and he didn't press me further. Years later, when I was diagnosed with PTSD, I'd tell him, and he'd come to understand.

Two decades after our acting class, even though we'd live over two thousand miles apart, we'd still be good friends. I think we always will be.

———

In graduate school, I lived in a three-bedroom apartment on the Allston/ Brighton border, down the block from Mr. T's, a pizzeria located at a street corner T stop, with two roommates: Josie, a restaurant manager, was dating a man who was arrested for (and eventually convicted of) conspiracy to commit murder; and Jeannie, a food addict, was in trouble with creditors who called our apartment all hours of the day and especially at 7 a.m. on Saturdays.

I paid my share of the bills on time and cleaned our bathroom weekly, but Josie and Jeannie, who were (respectively) five and seven years older than I was, sat me down to tell me that I was "an irresponsible child who contributes nothing" to the apartment. I didn't have any furniture to add to the décor and I couldn't buy any because I was living on a $500 per month fellowship stipend and student loans. Still, I thought they were right: I was unworthy.

On my birthday, Josie and Jeannie presented me with a cake and sang "Crappy Birthday to You." I smiled politely and thanked them for the celebration, silently harboring my hurt feelings. I expected to be treated poorly and questioned my negative reaction: Had they really behaved like jerks or was I being too sensitive? While I wanted better, I didn't know if I deserved better.

When Josie's boyfriend was out on bail, I was afraid for my safety when he came over for dinner and spent the night. My bedroom was a former sitting room with two French folding doors, no lock. I was afraid of being murdered while sleeping. Despite telling myself I was probably just being silly, I tied the doorknobs together with cord, an idea I thought of from watching *MacGyver*.

When I told my mother about Josie's boyfriend and mentioned that I'd accepted a few collect calls from the county jail (Josie had ordered that I must always accept), my mother didn't seem concerned. I used her reaction as a barometer for my own, as I had for my entire life. I thought perhaps my anxieties were unfounded.

I talked about the situation lightly with Daniel and Lauren. I thought using humor was more acceptable and more attractive than expressing my worry, or crying, which I frequently did in the shower. Daniel addressed my demeanor in his profile piece, an article he titled "Humor Is Everywhere":

"I'll laugh uncontrollably, and at other times I'm really scared to death,"
she confides to me, having erupted in a fit of laughter—nervous laughter, I
suspect—that turned her face red. "Sometimes I feel like people think I'm just
weird, because I have these weird stories. Sometimes I really wonder, these
people must think I'm crazy," she laments.

A nexis search reveals, however, that Strauss does indeed tell the truth. The
Boston Globe *reported on September 28 of last year that [Josie's boyfriend]*
was arrested for allegedly conspiring to murder the owner of a restaurant. He
was also arraigned for allegedly intimidating and bribing a witness who
planned to testify against him in court.

One day, at the start of our tutoring shift, I announced that Josie suspected that our phone was being tapped by the FBI. As I relayed the details, I was secretly conducting a reality check: If my listeners responded with concern, I'd know that my anxiety was warranted. If they brushed it off, I'd know I was overreacting.

Lauren's eyes went wide. Daniel sat up in his chair.

"What?" Daniel said. He let out a nervous laugh. "Are you kidding me?"

I continued: "There's this clicking on the line that we haven't heard before."

And Josie was suspicious of an unmarked car parked outside our building, which she believed was manned by a detective who was watching us. She said she thought the authorities believed her boyfriend was involved with the mob (this was before 9/11, when the biggest threats in Boston were Whitey Bulger and his comrades).

"You're going to school for screenwriting and you're living a movie-of-the-week!" Daniel exclaimed.

He made it sound as if I was special:

Her ability to overcome not only conspiracy to commit murder, but also a robbery at gunpoint the summer she worked as a cashier at CVS, as well as professors who she believes harass her, hints at a hidden reservoir of courage, strength, and humor. Her friends agree.

"People might almost be misled, because she might just sit there and be more quiet and on the sidelines, and you might miss out on a lot of things, because you don't get to know her," says Lauren Gaitley, Strauss' best friend in Boston. Rick Bow, Strauss' co-worker, concurs: "She's quiet at first, but she's a remarkably funny woman, once you get to know her."

When Daniel interviewed me, he asked me about my life, about where I'd grown up. I told him about my parents' divorce. He told me about how his father had died when he was in college and how he'd been stricken with clinical depression soon after. He lightened the mood by asking more about my roommate situation, about Josie's boyfriend. He called me "Agent Strauss." I called him "Agent Oxford." He seemed to have an affinity for me, as I had for him:

Strauss has the ability to use her experiences, however frightening, to further her career aspirations: to write for a television drama or sitcom, and to teach literature and film.

"It makes me more determined to get what I want," says Strauss, referring to the situation with [the alleged conspirator].

I believe her.

Later, he interviewed Lauren to ask her to provide further insight into my character for the profile piece. Lauren told me he asked her what kind of guy I wanted to date.

Daniel called me on the phone to follow up. "Agent Strauss," he began, and then asked me to go to a movie.

———————

"Ooooh," Josie and Jeannie said when they saw me getting ready.

"You look nice," Josie offered as I stood, wearing jeans and a sweater, in front of our full-length hallway mirror.

"Thanks," I said. I thought she might've meant it, too. I grabbed my apartment keys and put my hand on the door.

"Don't do anything I wouldn't do," Jeannie said, then looked at Josie and giggled.

"Don't wait up," I retorted, and left before they could respond.

Daniel picked me up and drove us to a movie theater in Chestnut Hill, where he paid for my ticket to *Liar Liar*, and bought a medium-sized popcorn for us to share. I thought this was a definite sign that he liked me as more than just a friend.

While we waited for the movie to start, Daniel joked and I laughed and joked back. I perceived our interaction as flirtatious. At one point, I touched his arm, to see how I'd feel.

I felt as if I could fall in love.

———————

After the movie, Daniel asked if I wanted to go out for dinner so that we could talk more. I thought maybe he was going to confess his feelings for me.

At our table for two at an empty Thai restaurant on Beacon Street, over plates of fried rice, Daniel and I talked about graduate school and the writing center and the premise of *Liar Liar*, about how great it would be to just tell everyone what you truly thought about them.

"So, Agent Strauss," Daniel said, pressing his lips together in a way that caused his dimples to spring into action on his cheeks. "What kind of person do you want to date?"

I felt my pulse quicken. I thought I knew where our conversation was going.

"Someone who's non-stalker-like," I began.

Daniel chuckled. He knew about Jack and Ray.

"Someone who has a good sense of humor," I continued, more seriously. "Someone who can have a meaningful conversation."

Daniel nodded. "Is there someone you have your eye on?"

My heart was pounding.

"Yes," I said.

"Yes?" he asked, leaning forward. He looked me in the eye and grinned. "Well, who is this guy? Tell me!"

I felt simultaneously enthralled and terrified. "You," I said.

"Oh," he said. His eyes left mine for the table.

I saw the waiter and busboy standing nearby, appearing to be listening.

"Oh no," I said, feeling my face flush. I suddenly wanted to run out of the restaurant. "This is so embarrassing."

"No," Daniel said. "Don't be embarrassed."

"Well, if you don't feel the same way," I began.

"I think you're a great person, Agent Strauss," Daniel said. "I think you're really cool. I admire you a lot. But after Marcia, dating is just too much. I can't do that now. I wish I could put it more eloquently, but I can't."

My face was burning. I looked into my water glass, wishing my feelings would wash away.

"You're blushing," Daniel said. "It's cute."

"So the interview was just an interview," I said. "And nothing more."

"Yes," Daniel said. "Look, I have clinical depression. I take medication. I don't feel like my true self. So I'd never be able to date you."

I didn't know whether he was trying to protect me from some inner demon or let himself off the hook with an excuse. Why had he asked Lauren what kind of guy I wanted to date? Why had he asked me? What was the movie and dinner invitation about, if it wasn't a romantic overture?

I'd made a mistake. I blamed myself: I'd dared to think I could have a guy I really liked as my boyfriend. I'd gotten it all wrong.

Daniel handed me a copy of the profile piece. There was an "A-" written at the top of the first page. "Dating Marcia made me realize who I really want to date," he said. "Someone nice, sweet, funny."

I'd once thought that someone could be me.

Daniel insisted on paying for dinner, and we left the restaurant. We were both quiet on the drive back to my brownstone. When we arrived at my building, I apologized. I had thought being honest and forthcoming about my feelings for Daniel would be a risk worth taking, but now I worried I'd jeopardized a friendship.

"I'm so embarrassed," I said, reaching to unhook my seatbelt, which, to my dismay, was stuck.

"Don't worry," Daniel said, keeping his eyes on the windshield. "I'll put it in the vault." He was quoting a line from "The Betrayal," a *Seinfeld* episode about secret keeping.

I wasn't sure I believed him.

I began to thrash around in my seat, trying to get the seatbelt loose. "I'm stuck," I said, starting to panic.

"What?" Daniel finally looked in my direction.

"The seatbelt," I said, pushing the release button again and again. "I can't get it to unlock."

"Uh-oh," Daniel said. "That happens sometimes. Press it again."

I did. Then Daniel tried. Finally, it unbuckled.

"You okay?" Daniel said.

I didn't know if he was referring to the seatbelt or our conversation. "I'm fine," I responded, and opened the door.

When I entered my apartment, I found Josie and Jeannie on the couch eating handfuls of M&Ms, their eyes glued to the television.

"How was your *date*?" Josie asked.

"Did he kiss you?" Jeannie inquired.

"Details, details!" Josie squealed.

I went to my room and cried. I called Lauren. "Better to find out now," she said.

My mother said the same thing when I told her a few days later. "What if you'd started having sex with him?" she asked.

What if I had? I thought silently, angrily. That's what couples did. *Would that have been so bad?*

I didn't understand why my mother had brought up sex. Daniel and I hadn't dated, and now we weren't going to. I knew that if Daniel and I became a couple that we'd become physical with each other. But for some reason I hadn't seen sex on the horizon. I hadn't gone that far in my mind. At the time, I wasn't aware of the way I was avoiding sex, even in terms of thinking about it. That was how I kept my past "in the vault."

After my date (or whatever it was) with Daniel, all night I tossed and turned, unable to sleep. I felt as if someone I loved had died. I'd fallen for Daniel. I'd fallen hard. And yet we'd never even started a romantic relationship, or kissed.

I didn't understand how it was that I'd developed such strong feelings for him, and yet the reality was that I had. Was I in love with the idea of being in love? I don't think so. I think what happened was that, for the first time, I opened my heart and I let a man in.

"Agent Strauss," Daniel wrote in navy blue ink at the bottom of my copy of his profile of me. "We live in a cynical world! ~ Agent Oxford."

———————

The following week, I overheard Daniel talking to one of the other writing center fellows about a new girlfriend, a classmate with voluptuous breasts. I internally deliberated Daniel's explanation as to why he couldn't date me. If he couldn't date me because of his clinical depression or the timing of his breakup with Marcia, why could he date this woman? I thought perhaps he'd rejected me because of me, because of my body. What I didn't think was that perhaps it wasn't about my perceived deficiencies but about Daniel's own human flaws.

Daniel sent an email saying he hoped I didn't "have any negative feelings" about what had happened between us. "We're cool," he wrote. "I realize, thinking back on it, that I may've sent mixed signals." He said he was sorry.

I didn't forgive him. I felt hurt. I responded by enumerating his mixed signals, as if to prove I'd been misled, that it wasn't all in my head. He replied to defend himself: He'd only been doing his job as a profile writer by asking the questions he had. The rest, he claimed, was just the usual interchanges and dialogue of friendship. It was nobody's fault, he concluded.

After that, he avoided me. I thought I'd handled the situation poorly and had ruined everything by expressing myself. When he saw me, he wouldn't look me in the eye. When he graduated, I heard he moved out of state. I thought I'd never see him again.

Almost ten years later, on Valentine's Day, I did.

I was on my way home after a long day of work, feeling self-piteously mournful and alone as a single woman amidst a crowd of couples holding hands and several men carrying bouquets of flowers and boxes of chocolate, en route, I imagined, to their lovers. I was walking past the Someday Café in Davis Square, Somerville, two blocks from where I lived, when I saw Daniel sitting at a table by the window, typing on a laptop.

I thought my mind was playing tricks on me. I stood for a moment, waiting to see if he might look up and recognize me, but he didn't lift his head. I thought about tapping on the window, but something stopped me.

I stood by the brick siding next to the window so that I could remain hidden as I peeked inside several times, as if through a looking glass, but still I couldn't confirm that he was Daniel.

I went home and changed into my pajamas, my usual post-work habit, and called Lauren. She told me I needed to get dressed and march back to the café and see if the man was Daniel. I had to go up to him and say hello. "You have to find out," she said.

I knew she was right. It was Valentine's Day. What if this was fate? My mind spun a romantic fantasy: What if we hadn't been ready for each other in graduate school, but now we were?

What was more the reality was this: I wasn't letting go of my past. I wished to make what had happened "unhappen," which was impossible, as well as symptomatic of my unresolved trauma. If I could change history, I believed, I wouldn't have to face my pain. Instead of accepting the way it was, mourning my losses, and moving forward, I remained stuck in a holding pattern, blindly keeping my (love) life stationary.

I put my work clothes back on, blotted my nose and forehead with face powder and my mouth with lipstick, returned to the café, and walked inside. The man I thought was Daniel was still there.

"Daniel?" I said, standing a few feet away.

He didn't seem to hear me. Or, I thought, perhaps it wasn't him, so hearing someone call "Daniel" meant nothing to his ears. I said his name again, louder. He didn't look up. I walked over and put my hand on his shoulder.

He turned toward me. Recognition washed over his face.

"Do you remember me?" I said at the same time he said, "Tracy?"

His face lit up. He stood, and we hugged.

"What're you doing here?" I asked as he sat back down.

"I just moved here," Daniel said.

"From where?" I asked.

He'd been in Texas, pursuing a master's in media studies, but he'd decided to drop out of the program to return to Boston.

"Do you want to sit down?" he asked.

I didn't want to let on that I didn't have plans for Valentine's Day. I didn't want Daniel to know that I was single, that I'd failed to find a life partner. I thought he'd take that information as confirmation that he'd made the right decision not to date me in graduate school. Perhaps he'd think I wasn't yet married because my character was too deficient for love. I didn't take into account that Daniel was sitting in a café by himself: He was likely also single.

"I can't stay," I said. "I have plans. But maybe we can meet up sometime?"

"That would be great," Daniel said. "Wow, I can't believe we ran into each other after all these years!"

A week later, when we met for coffee (well, tea for me—truth be told, I've never had a cup of coffee; I love the smell but not the taste), I asked Daniel about what had happened when we were in graduate school, when he wrote that profile of me, when we went out and he asked me about whom I wanted to date, and I revealed my feelings for him. I wanted to know what he was thinking. I wanted to understand.

He looked up at the ceiling for a moment as if he were trying to find the truth there, or (part of me wondered) the right line. "Honestly?" he finally said. "I don't remember that."

I wasn't sure I believed him.

"I have a bad memory," he continued. "I'm not saying it didn't happen the way you've said, I just don't remember it. It doesn't sound surprising though. A woman I knew in Texas said something similar about her experience with me."

He shrugged and smiled.

For the first time, I wondered what had attracted me to Daniel in graduate school, because now I didn't feel the same pull. At the café, he appeared worn. I could still see his charisma and the way his dimples danced around his cheeks, but, underneath that, I saw someone who wasn't being honest with himself, or with me. I wondered if he'd been that way in graduate school, too.

Was I making unfair assumptions?

"I'd really like to be friends," Daniel said. "Would you be up for that?"

I wasn't sure. But I'd grown a lot since graduate school, and I wanted to think that Daniel had as well. I wanted to give him a second chance.

I wanted to remain open. I didn't have many friends, especially straight guy friends. "Okay," I said. But I didn't have high expectations.

Although we were living in the same city, Daniel and I kept in touch mostly via Facebook status updates, or an occasional email, such as when I found out he'd donated to my fundraising efforts for the local rape crisis center and reached out to thank him for his benevolence. We rarely saw each other, except to attend two singles events together. I still felt a kinship with him, though that might've just been due to a shared history and social status rather than any deeper connection. At a synagogue mixer, we agreed to separate so as to leave ourselves open to finding "a match" among the other attendees, but we devised a code phrase for alerting one another if we needed rescuing from the presence of strangers: "These pretzels are making me thirsty" (of course, a famous line from a *Seinfeld* episode). Then, Daniel started what would become a serious long-term relationship with a woman he met online, and I didn't hear from him until after their breakup.

When Daniel attended my fortieth birthday party, my friend heard he was single and suggested we date. My friend and her husband thought we'd make a good couple.

"That's funny," said Daniel, before he quickly changed the subject.

CHAPTER 5
I WANT TO KNOW WHAT LOVE IS

Dear Future Life Partner,

For years, I yearned to know what love was. I bumbled around brainwashed by my family's definition, which stymied my love life. But I wasn't the only one struggling with the meaning of love. I think the men I met were, too.

I want to know what love is, with you.

How do you define love? How do we, as a couple, define it? What in your life has affected your ideas about love and how to find it?

I came to understand, slowly, that only in coming to terms with my past could I begin to listen to my own heart, instead of my parents' messages or society's stereotypical measure of success in love. Only through letting go of what I'd bought into could I learn to embrace my true self and find joy in a life that wasn't the traditional and socially expected path of marriage and kids in your twenties or thirties. So many of us don't fit into the mold we've been programmed to think of as "normal," but when things don't go according to the proverbial timeline, that doesn't mean there's anything wrong or deficient with us, or our love lives. When we've put ourselves out there for a long while, especially if we've been through rough times, we've gained the insight to reshape the definition of love and happiness, in a way that better serves us.

It's taken me years to get here. For so long, I didn't want to accept the truth of my absentee dating history, as if somehow I could go back and change facts, and, in effect, change where my love life ended up (not) going. Whenever I heard a love song on the radio, I mourned the common life experiences so many people sang about, so many human struggles and elations related to love, rites of passage I'd never lived and wondered if I ever would.

I had to leave behind my belief that I was an outsider in the world, my notion that I was for some reason barred from an aspect of life it seemed everyone else was privy to by nature of simply having been born. The reality is, so many of us are without a partner, by choice or not by choice, for reasons beyond our control: Everyday circumstances bring people together or draw us apart, teaching us about love—how we want to be loved, how we don't want to be loved, how we love others, why we love others, how others love us or don't love us, how we love ourselves or don't love ourselves. Dating has a lot to do with numbers and compatibility, random factors that aren't a reflection of our capability or our worthiness for finding a partner. But what is in our power, what we can do, is to prepare for ultimate success by examining what's shaped our concept of and approach to love in relationships, and seeing what, if anything, is in our way. In my case, I had to find the courage to face the false kind of love I'd grown up with, and how it had set me up for failure. Only then could I grieve the loss of time and the men I could've had relationships with but didn't. I had to clear out the toxicity in order to create space inside myself. Only then would I open the door to love. Only then was there room for the love of my life— you—to enter.

In the process, my world would turn upside down—or, more accurately (as I'd eventually come to realize), right side up.

Necessary Losses

AFTER GRADUATE SCHOOL, over a year passed before I met my next potential boyfriend, while working my first real job.

Six months after earning my master's degree, I left Boston for upstate New York to take a position in outreach and publications at my undergraduate alma mater. I'd considered moving out to Los Angeles to try to "make it" as a writer for a television series or to work for a film production team so that I could climb my way up a ladder I imagined would lead to a feature screenplay deal, fame and fortune and an Academy Award, or at least a stable job as a writer. While one of my college mentors called this "following your star," my mother referred to this as my impractical dream.

When I interviewed in Hollywood for a writer's assistant position at a well-known production company, a respected television drama series director asked what I wanted to do with my life. What was my professional goal?

"I want to write," I declared. "I want to share stories with the world." I wondered if that sounded cliché, or overly romantic, but it was my heart's pursuit and I felt a thrill finally saying it out loud.

To my dismay, the director said, "Go back to the east coast then. Don't work for me, or anyone out here, or you'll be at the office fifteen, sixteen hours a day plus weekends. You'll never write. You'll regret it. Go get yourself a nine-to-five job that pays your bills and doesn't suck the energy out of you and write."

At first, I thought he was just being polite so as to avoid telling me the hard truth of why he wasn't going to hire me as his writer's assistant. My past drove my self-critical thoughts: I wasn't "Hollywood" enough. I had frizzy ("ugly") instead of smooth and straight ("pretty") blonde hair, and my pale skin burned rather than tanned. I didn't have big enough breasts or cool-looking sunglasses. I wasn't worthy. I didn't belong. But the reality was that the director was speaking from a place of professional insight, consideration, and wisdom.

Admittedly, though I was disappointed, I was also relieved. I didn't know how I'd manage socially or financially in Hollywood. As my mother had said, it was an impractical dream. And so, I wouldn't apply for any more jobs there. When I informed my mother, she was glad.

"I wouldn't be able to handle it if you lived three thousand miles away," she said.

I felt myself bristle at her response. I didn't say so, but I felt confined by her wants, expectations, and rules, what I saw as her attempts to discourage me from pursuing my goals rather than helping me reach them. But I pushed my irritation aside, chalking up her behavior to a case of motherly overprotectiveness: She was saying such things out of experience and love. Or at least that's what she always told me. And I believed her.

I thought I instead might become a writing professor. In graduate school, along with tutoring in the writing center, I'd also been a teaching assistant and had enjoyed the role, but after graduation finding a full-time position was difficult. Ultimately, I was hired for two adjunct positions, one at a university in Rhode Island and the other at a community college on the north shore of Massachusetts. I didn't have a car, nor could I afford one. Every day, I commuted four to six hours by mass transit (depending on whether I just missed the connecting bus or train) while earning an unsustainable wage without health insurance. Every night, I came home exhausted and found Josie and Jeannie on the couch eating M&Ms and watching television. I didn't want to live with them any longer, but I didn't have the money to rent my own place, nor did I want to try living with different roommates, because I assumed they'd be just like Josie and Jeannie. When I looked at the few available studio apartments that I could hardly pay for, I saw that my budget would rent me nothing but a cramped room in a poorly managed and filthy building in a sketchy part of town. I didn't know of any resources out there that could aid me. Who would help me, financially or in other ways, until I got my life off the ground? My parents didn't offer. I could only depend upon myself

I felt trapped in a dead-end existence, desperately seeking a way out.

"We can think of no better person for the position," my future boss said over the phone.

I thanked my future boss but turned her down, even though I'd not only applied but I'd happily interviewed for the job, because I loved my alma mater. I felt safe there, protected in a way from the world. But I really wanted to stay in Boston. I wanted to build the life I dreamed of having in the city: I'd become a full-time professor, write screenplays or publish a novel, meet my life partner, get married, and have kids.

I said goodbye to my future boss and immediately called my mother to tell her about the offer and my decision. My mother promptly told me I'd made a mistake. She said I needed to be realistic. Was she right? The truth was I didn't have the financial ability to live in Boston. My mother said that sometimes what we want in life isn't possible. She said I should take the job, which would provide a steady income and benefits. She said I should hang up with her and call back my future boss right away, before it was too late.

"Just let go," my mother said, referring to my struggle (and my desire?) to make things work in Boston. "It'll be so easy."

I thought my mother knew more than I ever could about what was best for me, so I listened to her, instead of my heart. I accepted the job. I thought I'd feel better then, but I didn't. I'd made a choice from the perspective that I had no choice. I felt I'd lost my fight for the life I wanted and had instead surrendered to the life I believed I'd been dealt.

Three weeks later, I got into the back seat of a taxi to head to the airport, with my belongings piled at my feet. I turned to look out the rear window, fixing my gaze on the brownstone, the place where I'd resided for two-and-a-half years, where I'd hoped my life would begin, until the taxi turned the corner and I lost sight of it.

———————

Working at my alma mater provided stability. I established myself professionally and financially and started contributing to a retirement plan. I earned enough money to afford a car, which was a necessity where I lived, and I gained skills in writing, editing, and public relations. I enjoyed many of the duties of my job: writing and editing an alumni magazine, advising a student organization, and running a student-alumni career exploration program in Boston, New York, and Washington, D.C. The English department I'd studied in as a student allowed me to teach for them in the evenings, and I even devised and implemented a new course in screenwriting for the college, which built up my confidence as well as my resumé. I found that teaching was something I not only liked but loved. Teaching didn't feel like work. Like writing, it fed my soul. I began to think that maybe the kind of life I wanted was still attainable. It was just going to take me more time than I'd planned to achieve it.

My weekends were lonely. Living at the top of a hill that overlooked the alfalfa fields of a valley, I longed to return to the pulse of Beantown, the proximity to cafés and convenience stores, mass transit, people my age, and a vibrant literary community. I was twenty-five years old and living in a rural town where there seemed to be more cows than human beings. I was one of two people who wasn't a college student and who was under the age of thirty, a statistic I was provided by the only other person who fell into that category, a woman who'd been my classmate and who was working at the town planning office.

Socially isolating myself was easy. I could ignore the demons of my past that a relationship would require I face. But that didn't mean I was happy.

My job was based in the act of socializing, but in a business context and mostly long-distance, in writing, which was a more comfortable mode for me than face-to-face interpersonal interactions. I corresponded via email with Joey, an alumnus a year older than me (we'd never crossed paths as students), who lived in Los Angeles and worked for a production studio. Joey wrote his emails in all lowercase letters and often quoted Hunter S. Thompson. He told me I "intrigued" him. On my first day of teaching, he sent me flowers with a card that said, "You exist as inspiration, curiosity, and a link to the future come back from the past." He gave me hope. Like me, Joey dreamed of making it big in Hollywood. He talked about believing in second chances and having faith in your aspirations. When we were in touch, I felt alive.

When he took a trip to visit his family in Buffalo, he drove the distance to meet me in person. We ran like kids, with unbridled glee, through the campus and the hallways of his old dormitory. I brought him to my screenwriting class as a guest speaker. He chatted with my students about life in the "real world" of Hollywood. They loved him. I thought I might be starting to, too.

At the time, I wasn't aware that my concept of relationships and potential boyfriends was narrow-minded. In order to feel "comfortable" (read: "safe"), I had a particular set of requirements for a mate. He had to be educated, financially stable, physically fit, and a few inches taller than me. I wouldn't consider dating a man who was more than a few years older than I was, because I thought the dynamic would be one of sexual perversion; in my eyes, an older man was a predator to a younger woman. I also didn't date men who were younger, because I thought that would place me in the role of the predator. I never examined my preferences, I just knew I wouldn't and couldn't change them. I was even turned off by the idea of dating someone who looked older; balding men my age appeared to me as if they were middle-aged. I wasn't being vain; I was closing myself off to potential boyfriends by viewing men and relationships through the lens of my abusive past. I didn't really see what I was doing. I made decisions based upon my own outdated and unconscious trauma-informed definitions of danger and safety.

Joey was twenty-six and balding. I told myself to stop being so picky, but my negative association to his lack of hair nagged as I treated him to dinner at the Inn on Main Street to thank him for the time he'd taken to speak with my students. I was glad to be with a peer for the first time in a long while. After dinner, we walked to the campus lot where our cars were parked, and Joey asked if he could stay the night at my apartment. He said it was too late to drive back to Buffalo.

Part of me wanted to say yes but the rest of me froze, a nebulous fear reaching up through my throat, into my jaw, spreading across my tongue. My thoughts began to race. I searched my brain for a legitimate reason to say "no." I literally didn't think I could survive having a man stay overnight with me, though I couldn't say why.

It was 8:30 p.m. Buffalo was two hours away. I debated whether Joey really thought it was too late to make the trip, or if he was trying to trick me into sleeping with him. I imagined the scene: I'd let Joey stay on the futon in my living room. In the middle of the night, he'd creep into my bedroom, pull back the covers, and try to have sex with me. If I didn't want to, he'd either ridicule me or rape me. I berated myself for my suspicions—part of me really thought that Joey was a decent guy—but I was too afraid to test my sense of trust. I wasn't ready to cross the line between my own wish for a boyfriend and the reality of being seen by a man, both physically and emotionally, which would also entail me truly seeing myself.

I assumed Joey wanted casual sex rather than a caring relationship. Although I wished to be more easy-going, I wasn't into one-night stands. I thought that made me a prude. Within my mind echoed my father's voice, calling my mother "rigid" and telling me I was just like her. I was ashamed of my body and my fear.

Looking back, I can't say for sure that a one-night stand was what Joey wanted. But I didn't ask him to clarify his intentions, because I assumed I'd be derided for my way of thinking. I didn't know it at the time, but I was processing the present as if it were a scenario from my history.

"I really don't have a place for you to sleep," I said. "All I have is a futon."

I thought he'd drop it then.

"The futon will work," he said.

I thought I heard a pushy edge in his reply. In hindsight, I might understand the "pushy edge" as indicative of benign romantic interest, but back then I interpreted it as a predatory-like insistence and all I could hear was a girl's voice within me clamming up, begging *no, no no no no.*

"I'm sorry," I said more firmly. "We barely know each other. I don't let guys stay over until I know them better."

Joey's face appeared crestfallen. "But then I'll have to go to a hotel," he said.

There was a hotel a two-minute drive from campus. "I'm sorry," I said again, telling myself that his sleeping arrangements weren't my problem. I got into my car and pulled the seatbelt across my body.

Joey stood next to my opened door. He grinned and looked me in the eyes. "Are you sure?" he asked.

I unbuckled the seatbelt, got out of the car, and hugged him. "I'm sure," I said. "It was great meeting you. Really, it was. Thanks again for coming to my class." Then I got back into my car, shut the door, and drove away, feeling both relieved and disappointed.

I rarely heard from Joey after that, until I didn't hear from him at all. I felt sad that I'd passed up an opportunity for a potential boyfriend. I tried to convince myself that I'd made the right decision, and that I was better off without him.

I threw my attention into my job and my writing. I thought that if I could excel in my career I'd find greater life success: I'd be liked. In turn, I'd be loved. Consequently, I'd find you, my life partner.

I was deluding myself, digging my own kind of grave.

My job brought forth my unresolved dysfunction with authority figures and personal agency. I didn't realize it at the time, but my past shrouded my mental lens and colored my daily interactions. When my boss smiled, I saw the smile I'd learned to show as a child mirrored back at me, the kind that covers up your true thoughts and feelings.

In the beginning, my boss showered me with compliments, which made me uneasy. I didn't trust anything she said to be genuine. When my honeymoon period was over, her feedback became more pointed and picky.

When we hosted events, particularly off-campus, she told me I shouldn't eat because it gave the wrong impression to our constituents: Eating would make us look too casual, unprofessional. I was under the impression that she held herself to a higher standard and didn't eat before or afterward. Obedience was one of my strongest reflexes, and so, naturally, I followed suit. Some days, my boss jogged by the house where my apartment was located, as it was on her run route, and when I entered the office the following morning she commented on whether or not my car had been in the driveway. If it hadn't been, she asked where I'd been, what I'd been doing.

One day, she sat me down and said she'd made a decision: I wasn't to teach any more classes. "It gives off the wrong impression about your dedication to your day job," she said. She told me that if I wanted to get promoted I'd have to "eat and sleep" my job.

But classes were in the evenings, not during the workday, I protested. Still, she countered, my teaching was diverting my energy and attention away from the role I'd been hired to fulfill.

I thought maybe she was right. Maybe I'd been wrong—disloyal—to pursue the joy that teaching had brought me. I felt guilty, but I also felt angry. I *was* dedicated to my day job. I did good work. But I didn't want my position to define me, to become my whole existence. Through my eyes, my boss's decree was a projection of the way I felt my mother had tried to hold me back, how she didn't want me to go to Hollywood or stay in Boston, didn't want me to pursue my interests and goals, to live the life I wanted to live—to be *me*. I believed she created a mold for me, without my input or permission. I saw the mold, fashioned around her beliefs and rules, as meant to contain the person I was and shape me into the person she desired I be. It would be many years before I'd come to terms with my mother's ways; for now, the dynamic played out within my relationship with my boss. I worked to appease and please her, but I never felt I ever measured up to her expectations.

Every day, my boss appeared in my office doorway with the Job Manager in her hand, dangling it like a carrot. "What can we cross off the Job Manager?" she asked, placing it in front of me, leaning her elbows onto my desk and tapping her nails against the polished veneer.

The Job Manager was the day-by-day "to do" list, insistent and immovable in its tightly printed black grid. According to my boss, the Job Manager kept operations intact.

Created and maintained by my boss, the Job Manager was always keeping tabs. It was always on-guard, monitoring progress, machine-like, never tiring, never faltering, never relenting in its list of mandates: brainstorm invitation concept, write down ideas, discuss invitation concept, finalize invitation concept, design invitations, retrieve stationery from store room, print invitation draft, proof invitations, print invitation final copy, proof invitations x2, fill out print shop request, photocopy print shop request, send invitations to print shop. . . . When a project was physically completed, a review of outcomes began: what went well, what didn't, how could I work to make things better the next time?

On certain special days, such as Founders' Day or Alumni High Tea, the Job Manager expected tasks to be completed in five-to-fifteen-minute intervals. There was no lunch break listed. There was no time allotted for going to the bathroom. Across the hall was the stall and, while no one directly commented on who went in or for how long, throughout the day all took note.

To me, the Job Manager was a relentless micromanager. It pointed out, in stubborn silence, that I could never wipe the slate clean. Nothing was ever over and done with, because the Job Manager was never without its list of things to do. My boss said that no matter the task it could always be done, and it could always be done better.

The Job Manager was oppressively watchful, and I felt constantly under its thumb. When one duty was crossed off ("completed"), another one moved up in its place. Every day I'd wonder, what was the use of beginning if I could never finish? I was always on the verge of failure; I could never truly succeed. I berated myself—it was my own fault: I'd taken this job. I'd made my bed, and my sentence was to lie in it.

"You can cross this out," I pointed to the "begin deceased list" line for the Poinsettia Memorial Project, and then held my breath, waiting for my boss to question whether the task was really complete, which she often did. I assured her it was done.

"Perfect," she said, as precise as a surgeon with a scalpel.

Perfect: meaning "not lacking or faulty in any particular; the soundness and the excellence of every part, element, or quality of a thing, frequently as an unattainable or theoretical state." Perfect. That's what my boss said at my performance review: I was "perfect." But I didn't believe the assessment. If I were "perfect," why was it that I was always so far from it? I thought maybe my boss just enjoyed the way she could make the "perfect" consonants click from her lips and tongue. The sound was seductive.

As time went by, I began to wake up in the morning with a stiff neck and a tight jaw, and a sense of dread, a strange fear that I might die during the day, a type of panic attack I'd had before but wouldn't come to understand or name for many years to come. I developed trouble swallowing meals, particularly bulky foods such as bread and meat. I lost a lot of weight. I started running after work to try to purge my stress through exercise, or to outrun it. After, I'd go home, shower, and work on my novel, which I'd originally started to write as a screenplay until I realized the story was too interior-minded for the genre. I was crafting a narrative about a young woman who lived and worked in a rural town and who was very depressed, as I was. I listened to U2's "Bad" and Led Zeppelin's "Stairway to Heaven," over and over as I typed, feeling the depths of despair within me.

If I worked hard enough, I thought, I could climb out of my misery. Life would get better. Or at least, I thought, I'd feel better about it.

I never wrote beyond the first chapter of my novel. In truth, I was working on a memoir. I was writing about myself, but I was too afraid to face the truth. I thought the truth would kill me. I developed writer's block as a coping mechanism, a barrier to my pain.

But truth can be like the contents of a pressure cooker: The more you try to contain it, the more it bubbles up, spreads and expands, until there's no place else for it to go but out. Soon, something would prompt my truth to burst forth from its confines.

———————

Eight months into my job, the week John F. Kennedy Jr.'s plane disappeared off the coast of Massachusetts, my father was diagnosed with lung cancer. I had a dream about Senator Ted Kennedy crying and when I woke up early that Saturday morning and turned on the television I heard the news about the plane. My father had just had a rib and a quarter of a lung removed. He'd spend the next several months undergoing extensive chemotherapy and radiation.

That day, I had an appointment to get my hair cut at a salon on Main Street. As the stylist took the scissors to my head, I told him about my father. He said he was sorry. Later, I left his shop in a daze, barely feeling my feet on the pavement. I couldn't stop thinking about my father, wondering when he was going to die. To tell the truth, I wanted him to die sooner rather than later. I felt as if he was bringing me down into the grave with him. I couldn't say why. I just wanted him to die so that I could live.

My thoughts troubled me as the heat and humidity swelled about my body. I felt disoriented, as if I was no longer of this world. I wondered if I ever had been. I decided to go to the Wegman's supermarket in town for the coolness of its air conditioning (I didn't have such an amenity in my apartment), where I could buy a muffin and a magazine. I went to Wegman's whenever I felt alone. Being around other people gave me the illusion that I was part of a group, a family—I belonged somewhere.

Wegman's was one of the more popular attractions in the rural area where I resided. Carloads of people, mostly local farmers and their wives, or young families who lived in mobile homes, traveled from miles and miles away and filled the aisles every Saturday and Sunday. One could eat breakfast, lunch, and dinner right in the store, and in between meals there was the Walmart to explore less than a hundred feet away. One could get a corndog there for a dollar-fifty, not that I ever did. Really what brought people to the locale, I thought, was the beautiful valley—in the words of John Keats, "Beauty is truth, truth beauty,— that is all / Ye know on earth, and all ye need to know"—where the land beckoned like the opened palm of a hand.

In the days following my father's diagnosis, I returned to Wegman's often, spending most of my time at the periodicals display, taking in the headlines: "John F. Kennedy Jr. Plane Lost"; "Routine Flight Goes Awry"; "JFK Jr. Feared Missing, Presumed Dead." I stood there, staring at JFK Jr. on a glossy magazine cover: the philanthropic brown eyes, the groomed brows full and dark like mindful caterpillars, the dashing grin—all pronounced dead before the person they were a part of had been found. His fate had been decided for him.

I felt forlorn, and angry.

I studied JFK Jr.'s face. He was wearing a lot of makeup, a creamy foundation. I wondered, had anyone ever seen what was underneath? The issue mesmerized me, churned inside my heart, tossed and turned, ruffled and agitated like rough seas. I couldn't stop my thoughts from coming, crashing forth like the tide. The events drew me in:

The plane had disappeared from radar and had plunged into the foggy depths of America's collective mind, the remains thought to be mixing with the waves that crashed and lapped in comfortable cyclical motions, gentle as a baby rocked, beside the shores of Massachusetts. According to article after article, John F. Kennedy Jr., his wife Carolyn Bessette, and her sister had not yet been found in the flesh. Still, the headlines confirmed: Hope was gone. The perfect couple had lost their lives. Yet were they really so perfect or was that a false perception that the universe had manufactured only to now destroy it by unveiling the truth?

Within a week, their bodies were found and authorities concluded that the plane crashed due to the pilot's loss of his visual sense of the horizon. Spatial disorientation is a killer.

What do you do when you suddenly no longer know which way is up? How do you re-orient yourself? Is it possible to save yourself, your life?

When I visited my father a few weeks after his diagnosis, I asked if he had a will. We were at the food court at LaGuardia Airport. He was enjoying the sugar on top of a cinnamon bun, which my father said he shouldn't have been eating, because sugar feeds cancer cells. I was sitting across from him, waiting for my flight, watching, wondering: I wanted to know my father's wishes, for his future, for his past, for his life, for his death, for me, about me, in relation to us. I wanted to know, before it was too late. I wanted to have an understanding. I wanted him to understand me, too.

He was thin because of the chemotherapy. He was telling me he'd lost six pounds because he wasn't eating very much, he wasn't very hungry, he was wasting away. I wanted to tell him I'd lost weight too, but I didn't say it. I figured he'd see it himself if it was noticeable, if it was anything. He should see these things. After all, I thought, he was my father.

When I asked him if he had a will, he didn't look up at me. He shook his head, no. "I had one when I was married to your mother, but I don't have a current one," he said. He wasn't paying attention to me. He was preoccupied with the food. "Why? Are there particular personal effects you want?"

His question took me off-guard. "All I want is you," I said. I was grasping for a father who wasn't there, who didn't exist.

He replied like the Cookie Monster, to the food in his hand, "Goooood," and then to me: "You want some?"

"No, thank you," I said. "I'm not hungry."

Back at work, my anxiety worsened, and so did my eating. I felt as if my body and mind were out of my control. I needed help. My mother said being anxious about my father's illness was normal—she understood, after all, as her father had died of cancer when she was close to my age. But more, she was very upset that I was unhappy at my job—she just wanted me to be *happy*, she said, her voice sharp with frustration. She suggested I see a therapist.

I went to the only mental health services center I could find within a twenty-five-mile radius, the Life Choice County Clinic which sounded more like a place where people had abortions rather than where they had their heads shrunk, though to me the concept was the same: insides severed and removed, disposed of, expunged. I was there to have my thoughts terminated.

I started seeing Bea, a middle-aged social worker, because I wanted to resolve my problems, but also because doing so pleased my mother. My mother wanted to hear the contents of my sessions. She asked me what I talked about in my meetings with Bea, and what Bea said in response. I reported the details, telling her much more than I wanted to share, ignoring my discomfort at such disclosure, because I thought my mother's need to know everything was paramount. My mother responded to my recaps by saying, "You have a lot more going for you than most people your age," but I wasn't convinced. She told me I had high self-esteem, though I didn't think that was true. I didn't object to her statements aloud, because I was confused about who was actually right: my mother or myself. When she visited, I asked her if she thought I looked thin and she said, "You look fine." When we went to a restaurant and I had trouble ingesting my meal, she became bothered: "It's like you're punishing yourself!" Over the phone she said angrily, "You know, you make it really difficult for people to help you," as if it were my fault. I wanted her to understand and accept me, but instead she took everything I thought or felt or did as if it were a personal affront.

The clinic was located within walking distance of campus and I was afraid someone who knew me might see me and report such a sighting back to my boss, so I went to my weekly appointments as surreptitiously as I could during my lunch hour.

The foyer served as a cramped waiting area. There was no receptionist. I sat in a chair beside a corner table covered with magazines, crossed my legs, and swished my foot from side to side, feeling increasingly impatient while I waited for Bea, who was always running late with her previous client. Above, on the wall, was a framed portrait labeled "Holy Mary, Mother of God." I read it as a swear phrase. I was living in a pervasively Christian community. I was pretty sure that Jewish the vicinity. The nearest synagogue was almost an hour's away, while this town had a church on almost every corner.

Bea to me talk about my job stress, my father's cancer, and my parents. I never went any further than that, and Bea never pushed.

_____

About after forty percent of my father's left lung was removed and labeled malignant, four months after he confirmed himself cancer-free, I was running, listening to the oldies station, the only station I could access on my radio Walkman. Radio reception was near absent in the depths of the valley, where the track was located, beside the alfalfa fields.

I was jogging to the rhythm of the music, my lungs taking in the air and letting it go. The breeze was picking up when a large shadowy man parked his red pickup truck and got out of the vehicle, unleashing a big black dog. The animal began to gallop fast, faster, faster, toward me. I stopped breathing, freezing for a moment, cold in my tracks: It was coming right at me, a pulsating fear washing over me like an ocean wave—*Lord have mercy on the boy from down in the boondocks.*

The dog turned, his black coat shining with a sense of urgency: *Go home.* I had to go home.

When I reached my apartment, I found my answering machine flashing. There was a message from Russell. I'd missed his call by ten minutes.

"Tracy," he began, "Dad got in a bit of trouble today. He's okay for now, but he had to have some emergency surgery on his brain. Call me."

I hadn't yet caught my breath as I dialed Russell's number. He didn't answer. I dialed my father's number so that I could speak with Donna, my father's girlfriend. My father had met Donna on the Long Island Rail Road, he said, it must've been fate, she'd changed his life. I'd assumed they'd met after my father left the house. But my mother told me that she knew Donna, had met her at one of my father's office functions years before. When I asked if she thought he'd had an affair, she quickly and curtly said, "No." I didn't believe her.

"Your father—" Donna's voice stalled, like a motor, after the initial greeting, coughed like a carburetor. "He—"

"What?" I prodded. My own question stopped my breath: Was he dead?

"He started not feeling well," Donna said. "He had a migraine, and eventually the pain got so bad he collapsed. I had to take him to the hospital in the middle of the night. He passed out in the car. The doctor says it was a tumor that bled on itself." She'd called Russell to tell him.

"But I just spoke with him the other day and he was fine," I said. "When did this begin?" I wasn't focusing: The words were a dust storm in my mind, the meanings caught in my mouth. I already knew the pain had begun months ago. My father had mentioned the headaches several times when we talked by phone, but he'd ignored the signs: The cancer had traveled to his brain.

"Two days ago," Donna said.

"Why didn't anyone call me *then*?" I asked. My heart began to pound against my ribcage as if it were trying to break out of a prison: hard, hard, hard, I thought I might die slow, slow, slow. I thought my heart might cease to beat at any moment.

"Oh Tracy, don't you give me that," Donna said. "There were other people who were more important than you to call."

"But I'm his daughter." I heard my voice sounding small.

"Well then you ought to act like one," Donna's voice escalated. "You're never here when he's sick. You're only around when he's well. Some daughter you are, he might be paralyzed and I don't think I can deal with taking care of that for the rest of my life!"

The words, these price tags of love, lingered in the air between us.

From the day Donna and I first met, when I was twenty and my father introduced me to her over egg rolls and Wonton soup and sesame chicken with rice at a Chinese restaurant just a few months after he moved out of the house, I knew she disliked me. I probably gave off a defensive vibe; after all, I was uncomfortable with the idea that my father was dating so soon after leaving my mother, and I felt as if I was betraying my mother by having dinner with my father and this woman he was sleeping with. I sensed that Donna saw me as an extension of my mother (my parents' friends had always said how much my mother and I looked and sounded the same) or as "the other woman," competition for my father's attention. I didn't find her to be very warm, or friendly. She flipped her long platinum-dyed hair as if to swat a fly. She wore a forced smile, a thick coat of mascara, and heavy red lipstick. She asked me about my major in college and what kind of writing I liked to do, then turned the focus onto herself and her myriad professional accomplishments. I tried to show her I was impressed by nodding, saying "wow" a lot, and asking follow-up questions, but she never warmed up. She complained about her boss, and then she and my father spent the rest of dinner making fun of her coworkers' bodies and personalities. When I didn't laugh, Donna gave me an icy stare.

Over the phone, she was unforgiving.

"I want to speak with my father," I said. The backs of my thighs were shaking, and my hands and my neck felt clammy. "What's the number for the hospital?"

"I don't know," Donna's voice scattered like dandelion seeds.

"I want to speak with my father," I said it again. My ear ached as I pressed it against the receiver.

"You *can't*," Donna's voice pushed against me, bruising, like an admonishment. "He's not able to speak with you right now."

"Well, his doctor, then," I said.

"Don't you dare call his doctor," she said. Her voice sounded like a growl now. Her words bit. "The last time you did that you really embarrassed us."

I'd spoken to my father's doctor after his original lung surgery, when he was unconscious, to hear an update. I'd called the hospital and told them I was his daughter and asked about his status and they put the doctor on the phone.

"But I'm his daughter," I said again, the word "embarrassed" sticking to me like glue. "I have a right to know what's happening to my father, to hear the truth."

"The truth," Donna's voice turned cold, "is that if your father knew how you really are, how you are treating me, he'd be very disappointed in you. In fact, I know he already is."

I shrunk back like a turtle. "This isn't the time to be discussing this," I heard my voice outside myself. "Right now my father is the issue."

My tongue was flypaper, thick and numb and sticky, and too big for my mouth, for speaking. I hung up the phone and took off my sneakers and clothes and got into the shower and stayed there for a long time, letting the sobs go as silently as I could so that no one would hear me or know what I thought or how I felt, my tears indistinguishable from the pin-needled stream, the rushing sound of the water.

Vigilance: That night an old ritual took over—my body's, my mind's—of not sleeping. I was like a little girl, afraid of the dark, afraid of the big monster under my bed, hiding in the shadow in the hallway, lurking in the darkness, waiting for the precise moment to spring on me. I remained on guard with fear as my cloak. My eyes remained stuck open, on the watch, unblinking, until eventually, after several hours passed, my lids grew too heavy to support. Finally, I let my body give in, let the dark heaviness take over, and, consumed with restless slumber, I closed my eyes.

I began to have a recurring dream in which I felt an uncensored and pervasive sense of impending disaster. I was in the passenger's seat of a car. My father was behind the wheel, driving, despite a blind spot, vision damage caused by the location of his brain tumor. "I don't have vision problems," he said. "My eyes are fine, it's my brain that isn't getting the message."

On a curve in the road, my father lost control of the car. There was a slow-motion skid and then we crashed. I felt myself dying. I heard a voice—it sounded like my mother's—saying "oh no," with sheer morbidity. Then it was over.

I imagined that when the tumor came apart in my father's brain it was like a malfunctioning plane's explosion: first the dull headache and nausea from the drop in altitude, then the disorientation, the pounding, the force of gravity taking over, the body's tumultuous plummet, down, down, breaking through the invisible shield, leaking a bloody red fire, the interior bursting through the exterior, nothing and no one salvageable. As a word, gravity is a close cousin to "grave." Meaning: serious, weighty, like tired eyelids. His condition was grave. Grave: a place of burial.

My father had survived the emergency surgery, but the long-term prognosis didn't look favorable, though that was only what I thought, not what my father would later tell me. *I'm fine*, he'd say. But what I heard from my father and what I held in my heart were separate entities at odds with each other, in conflict, diverging.

This made my mind run and my heart race.

I waited two weeks before visiting my father, despite suggestions from colleagues to go right away in case he didn't make it. I felt a deep reluctance to see him, for reasons I reflexively pushed away before I could even know them. However, I called the nurse to ask his status and I tried to reach him by phone. It was a couple of days before he was able to talk from his hospital bed. He told me that he saw the Grim Reaper standing in the doorway, "You know, with the cape and the scythe?" he said. "He just stood there, and then he left."

What he said frightened me. If my father could ward off Death, then he was more powerful than I'd ever thought.

Soon after, I terminated therapy.

As I sat in the waiting area before my appointment, I heard voices—Bea and her client—as if I were in the therapy room with them. Bea had forgotten to turn on the white noise machine, the little contraption that emitted sounds like waves crashing, so that those in the waiting area wouldn't hear what was spoken in confidence, for protection of privacy. For some reason, Bea kept the white noise machine inside her office instead of out in the waiting area, so I could do nothing about it. I was furious that she forgot. I could hear everything that was said, even though I didn't try to and didn't want to listen. I was unwillingly involved. I felt as if I was simultaneously the violator and the violated.

"I was nine years old," said the client, a young woman, "and she kept telling me the details of how she had sex with these men."

"Your mother?" asked Bea.

"Yes." The client was weeping. "I mean, I didn't want to hear it."

"That's a lot for a nine-year-old to handle," Bea cooed.

"When I have sex, I don't have an orgasm," said the client.

"When you had sex with Johnny, did you have an orgasm?" Bea asked.

The client hiccupped with sobs, "No-o-o-o."

I prayed the client wasn't a student at the college, though who else would it be? I didn't want to meet her eyes when she came out of the session. I didn't want to risk her recognition of me. How would it look to the student to see me, a staff person, there? The news would get around that I was unstable, unfit to perform my job. Ultimately, the client dashed from the session room, blinded by tears, and I went unnoticed.

When I walked into the office, I told Bea I wouldn't be coming back. This would be my final session, I told her, because nothing had changed in my life though I had talked and talked and talked in my sessions with her about my work stress and my father's cancer and my secret wish for him to die—I'd felt the loss of him years ago, I'd admitted, though I couldn't put my finger on why.

I hadn't yet allowed myself to know of the extensive sexual abuse I'd experienced as a child; I didn't let the few surface incidents I'd consciously retained enter my mind when I talked with Bea. But when my father got sick I felt as if

I went down some rabbit hole and I couldn't seem to find my way out. I didn't know if there even was a way out. Talking with Bea hadn't fixed my problems.

Many times, I'd asked Bea if, in her opinion, I had an eating disorder, but she would just shake her head no, I didn't starve myself, binge, or purge, did I? I didn't obsess about my weight, did I? I didn't have a warped sense of body image, did I? What I had was anxiety, perhaps a phobia, nothing a pill or two wouldn't solve, if I would just let a doctor give me a prescription, if I would just try that route, if I would just *trust*, have a little faith, that was my problem, she said. I not only refused the pills, but I had not broken down during any of my sessions, why was that, Bea demanded, and what was I hiding?

I'd failed the mental health litmus test: tears.

Now, I gathered my things.

"You're one of the most straightforward people I know," Bea said, surprising me with her statement. I wondered if she was being truthful or if she was simply trying to lure me to stay.

I stood to leave.

Bea's last words to me were that she had two wishes: that I stop battling my feelings and that I start to think about my thoughts regarding relationships with men. Sex.

I felt an electric charge zip through my body. I turned and walked out the door.

If You're Gone

I DIDN'T KNOW it then, but quitting therapy wouldn't solve anything. It would only indefinitely stall my life. I felt defeated by events that I believed had marred my ability to love and be loved. I didn't yet know that I could learn how to release the hold my demons had on my heart. I didn't yet understand that taking a leap of faith to face my ingrained destructive beliefs and habits could transform my pain and allow me to find and experience a meaningful relationship on my own terms. The more I worked to contain and forget my formidable past, the more my unspeakable truth had control over my life.

When I was twenty-six, I had a crush on my dentist.

I preferred to think that Dr. Mohgart was really named Bogart. Once aggravated by his dental sarcasm, I changed my mind about him while under the influence of the nitrous oxide. He was tall and tan and blond and forty-five and married with three teenaged children. In my head, I asked him to elope with me. I imagined he'd whisk me away from my life's chaos.

"There are risks in undergoing this procedure," Dr. Bogart said. "Nerve damage, loss of feeling, even death can occur."

I was lying there awake, under the knife, my body full-length on the chair, head and shoulders tilted behind me, almost like a back bend, my neck elongated like an ostrich's, the nitrous oxide turned on. My wisdom teeth were like cranky children, digging their heels in, refusing to let go. They were hidden under my gums and fused to my jawbone. In pulling them out, there was a lot of drilling and excavating, as if through cement. It was a horrible mangled mess of blood and bone and gum tissue.

Dr. Bogart had a strategy to the extraction, approaching each tooth with deft attention and care, with an intimacy and an intensity, as if he were making love.

When it was over, he gave me my teeth, two at a time, the pairs wrapped in a mound of gauze. "You can keep them," he said.

I uncovered the four fossils, my bones, and held them in the palm of my hand. They were oddly shaped, I thought as I stared, these hooked roots of spiraled corpses. The dead ends were stained a brownish-red. I saw them as a family of four: gone. And yet there I was holding them together in my grasp.

Within two days of the oral surgery, I was back in the office with my bottle of painkillers in my purse. Unable to tolerate the stress of the Job Manager, I made a work-related excuse to leave the office for an errand across campus—I had to drop off a form, or something, I said—so that I could visit the English department on the top floor of the ivy-covered academic hall. There, I tried to envelop myself in the quietude of the empty hallway. I looked at my former professors' names on their office doors, taking several slow breaths, sipping the air of literary contemplation, that same old clay and book smell from my days as a student, which wafted through the air with a calming sense of stability.

Dr. Bob Devlin, the chairman of the English department, emerged from his office to say hello. When I first started my professional position at the school, he told me to "please call me Bob" instead of "Dr. Devlin"—"We're colleagues now," he said. I felt funny at first, but I liked the way such a gesture felt respectful and inclusive.

A year older than my father, Bob lived in town with his wife and had two grown children, including a daughter who was a year older than I was. As a student, I never took any of Bob's classes, because his appearance scared me. He taught medieval literature, including *Beowulf* and Dante's *Inferno*. To me, he looked like Beowulf, or at least how I imagined Beowulf looked: scarily intense, with messy hair. I heard that Bob enjoyed discussing smutty topics, such as the works of Chaucer, at length, and that he was easily ticked off. He was also known for removing his shoes and socks and picking his toes in class. I once walked by his classroom and saw.

"I'm going to lunch," Bob said. "Would you like to join me?"

My thoughts began to race: Why did he want to have lunch with me? What did he want? "I'm sorry, I can't," I responded, feeling my face burn, trying to hide that. "I have to get back to the office." I looked at my watch as if to confirm with evidence, as if I couldn't do anything about it.

Bob nodded, looked at the floor, and then walked back into his office. I felt sorry.

Mary, the department secretary, took me aside. "Bob's one of the good guys," she said.

A few days later, I agreed to go to lunch with him at the diner on Main Street where all the townies hung out. I used to go there with my friends when we were students; we'd get the grilled cheese sandwiches and French fries and cokes and poke fun at the townies and ponder how anyone could actually live there for real, as if we were immune to the possibility of such circumstances.

The waitress came over. Bob asked what I was having.

"I'll have the chicken soup," I said. "And a glass of water."

"I think I'll have that, too," Bob said. "And a half a tuna sandwich with tomato, on rye."

We sat there in silence for a long while.

When the food arrived, I was aware of Bob's gaze as he watched me stir my soup, eat a half a spoonful, and then pour the broth over the vegetables, as if I were watering a garden.

"I just had my wisdom teeth out," I explained. "I'm not supposed to have anything too hard to eat."

Bob didn't reply. In fact, he didn't say anything at all, he just observed. He sat there in utter quiet, which unnerved me. I wondered what he was thinking, if it was about me, if it was bad. I assumed it was so. He slurped his soup, lifting brimming spoonful after spoonful into his mouth with a rhythm and pace that pleased him. He didn't care if he was messy or neat. He was one with the soup. The same was true with his sandwich. I envied him. He was there in the moment, enjoying this intake, all the disparate elements merging together, meshing textures and tastes. His cheeks bubbled with air as he let out a few burps, satisfied, making room for more.

I was hungry, but I was too afraid I'd choke if I took in anything else. I put my spoon down. I placed my water glass, which was large and red, in front of the bowl so that the uneaten part of the soup would be hidden from Bob's view. He looked at me briefly, then back down at his empty plate and bowl. I wondered why he chose to sit with me, why he wanted to have lunch with me, what he wanted in return. I was worried I'd have nothing to give. I placed my hands around the red water glass, my fingertips rubbing the mottled surface in a way that soothed my nerves.

Bob lifted his arm over my red glass of water and pointed with his finger into my soup bowl, at the uneaten food: "Is that because of your teeth or because of your life?" he asked.

I didn't expect his voice to sound so gentle.

"My teeth," I sputtered, looking away quickly but not before I noticed his eyes, soft brown circles that penetrated like darts of clarity. He knew. There was nowhere, no way, to hide. I had to admit the truth. How quickly things turned. How quietly I said it: "Because of my life."

Then I was overtaken by his eyes, which were laden with a kind of care I felt I hadn't earned. His eyes were probing, seeming to want to see through me, beyond words. My own eyes lowered to the table and stuck there.

"I'm sorry," I said. "I'm sorry."

I couldn't look at him. I thought that if he really knew who I was and what I thought, he'd want nothing to do with me. He bowed his head, as if he was praying, or, I thought, as if he were trying to latch himself into my eye line. I was too ashamed to look up at first, but something inside myself, or perhaps it was outside myself, like a force—faith—prompted me and I glanced up, for a breath. Bob seemed satisfied: "Okay," he answered softly, sitting back in his chair, pensively. "Okay."

Then there was so much to say that I couldn't say anything at all. My voice was caught in my throat like an animal in a barbed wire fence.

Bob's eyes flickered at me, large and intense, like an owl's. His were eyes that saw through darkness, without judgment. They upheld truth and held up my fear, to the light.

Outside, the rain had begun to fall, hard, needled drops pouring forth on the pavement, overwhelming the streets, rushing all at once to the windowsill, streaking the pane like tear stains. Inside, there was the fluorescent light illuminating the table, the pushing back of a chair, the clatter of the soup spoon on the saucer as the waitress took away what was left unfinished.

Bob didn't know the extent of my issues, because I didn't reveal them. He believed I had depression and gave me the name of a psychiatrist he knew, Dr. V., whose office was in the city, a forty-five-minute drive from where I lived in the valley.

When I told my mother I was going to therapy again, she was pleased.

I went to my appointments with the diligence of a "good girl," going through the motions in order to feel better, as if this course of counseling would be a prescriptive cure, especially since Dr. V. came recommended by the chairman of a college English department. I told Dr. V. that, while I understood he was a psychiatrist, I wasn't interested in taking any medication, because I didn't want any chemicals controlling my mind. At the time, I saw medication as a sign of failure, a belief I'd gotten from my mother. My mother disapproved of the use of antidepressants, stating they were a "crutch" that didn't solve one's problems; she said taking them was a sign of inner weakness. I believed her. I told Dr. V. that I was only interested in talk therapy. He said that was fine. Before each session, I wrote an outline and memorized the points I intended to cover.

Dr. V.'s office was located on the first floor of his house. With its separate entranceway, the office was carpeted and dimly lit. Unlike Bea's bare bones setup, Dr. V. had a traditional black leather psychoanalysis couch, the sight of which made me anxious. I sat upright in a wooden chair and Dr. V. sat across from me, beside a wall of books. I liked to look over his shoulder, out the window, at my sky-blue Honda Civic parked at the curb.

Dr. V. didn't ask many questions. He mostly sat still, waiting for me to speak, looking bored. My mother said this was a therapist's way of "drawing out the truth."

"I thought Dr. Tetley was bored sometimes," she added, as if to normalize my experience.

I thought Dr. V. didn't really care.

Similar to my time with Bea, I never cried in front of Dr. V., though I did see him more frequently than Bea, twice a week, because he was a doctor (and therefore I thought he must be better than Bea), because I thought more frequent sessions might solve my problems more quickly, and because my attendance made my mother feel less upset, which meant our phone conversations were less stressful for me.

One day, I brought along the lyrics to the song "If You're Gone," by Matchbox Twenty. I told Dr. V. that every time I heard it on the radio, I felt the song expressed my sadness about my father.

"It's written to a lover," Dr. V. said.

I suddenly felt my whole body burn. "Yes," I concurred but quickly brushed the association aside. "But more generally it's about losing someone you love. That's what I meant."

Dr. V. was a psychiatrist; he was an expert on what Freud had said about little girls and their fathers. But my attunement to the song was about more than Freud's theories of child development. Looking back, I'm not sure whether Dr. V. suspected that the song pointed to a trauma I'd long ago buried.

I never said another word about the song to Dr. V. and neither did he.

In fact, this was one of my last sessions with Dr. V., because I was unexpectedly hired as a writer at a Boston-area college, and I was about to leave upstate New York for good. I was moving back to Beantown, and I was ecstatic. When I asked for a referral for a therapist whom I might see in the Boston area, Dr. V. said, "I think you'll be fine without therapy." I wasn't sure if what he said was true, but I hoped that maybe being back in my element, in Boston, the city of my dreams, would be all I needed to fix my problems. I pressed Dr. V. for a name "just in case," but he said he didn't know anyone in Boston, because "there isn't much of a mental health community there."

I believed him.

Within a year of my moving into a studio apartment in Somerville, a city just north of Boston, my anxiety became too much for me to handle. I had frequent and severe panic attacks while driving to my job where my verbally abusive male boss was running several coworkers out of the office on a daily basis. I began suffering from debilitating bilateral arm pain that made it brutal to work on the computer at my desk; eventually, turning the key in my car's ignition switch to drive to my job was too painful. I spent my evenings and weekends alone and depressed, in bed with a migraine. Money was very tight. I brought a calculator to the supermarket and added up my items aisle by aisle, putting back what I couldn't afford, skimping on meals. I was still having trouble swallowing food and I remained underweight, though I made sure I never went below 110 pounds, which I considered an "okay" number ("normal" weight for my height and frame is 125–130 pounds). I knew I needed help. I phoned Dr. V. and asked if we could have phone sessions until I found a new therapist. He agreed and said he'd call me back in a couple of days to schedule an appointment, but then he never called back and he didn't return my follow-up messages.

I strongly preferred to see a woman practitioner, so I phoned twenty-five female providers using my insurance company's behavioral health list, but they all said they weren't taking on any new clients or they didn't accept my partic-ular insurance and I couldn't afford to pay out-of-pocket, or they didn't return my call. I felt worse and worse. After over a month of attempts, I realized my options were to either check myself into an emergency room or try a male ther-apist. I looked at a list of male therapist names. I'd liked the character "Dr. Ross" on the television series *ER*, so I took the risk and dialed the number of a therapist with the last name "Ross." His voice sounded friendly on the answer-ing machine, so I left a message. He called me back within a couple of hours and told me he was about to leave for a week-long vacation, but that he could see me when he returned. I asked him if he might have an associate I could see, because I really needed to see someone right away. In response, he offered me an appoint-ment for the next morning.

Dr. Ross wasn't a medical doctor; he was a psychologist with a PhD, yet I called him "Dr. Ross" instead of using his first name because he was old enough to be my father and I didn't want things between us to be too casual, familiar.

When I arrived for my first appointment, Dr. Ross appeared at the top of the office building stairs, tall and balding with glasses, a combination of brainy and athletic. His arm stretched downward to greet me in the foyer, like a rope over the edge of a cliff.

I took his hand and climbed upward.

Inside his small corner office, Dr. Ross sat on a black leather chair with his feet up on a matching ottoman. I sat across from him in a cushioned maroon fabric swivel chair closest to a bookcase and farthest from the window, because I didn't want anyone outside to catch sight of me.

Over the next weeks and months, before my sessions I memorized a list of thoughts I'd present about my anxiety and depression, my parents' divorce, my verbally abusive boss, the fact that I wanted to have a boyfriend but wasn't dating. I tried to control the agenda.

"I can't tell what you're feeling," Dr. Ross said, noting that my face was always expressionless. "You talk about such painful things, but you never cry."

"I cry," I said defensively. "In private."

"It might help to cry while you're here with me," he said. "You might feel better."

I didn't think so.

"Why not?" he gently inquired.

I told him about a recurring incident from my childhood.

On family vacations to the east end of Long Island, while my father drove our car he watched me in the rear-view mirror. On Old Montauk Highway, he accelerated up and down a stretch of steep hills as if we were at the beach riding the waves, only this was the road, not the ocean. With each tarred drop, my stomach fell, making me feel sick and sad and mad and scared.

When I asked my father to stop driving so fast, he laughed. I met his gaze in the mirror. His blue irises turned hard. He said, "Beg me."

My emotions were under my father's microscope, smeared on a glass slide. He got a thrill out of studying me.

Please, I tried. I was six, seven, eight, nine, and ten years old. *Please stop.*

He didn't stop until I cried.

I read *The Sociopath Next Door*, by Martha Stout, PhD. I saw it on Dr. Ross's office bookshelf and was mesmerized by the cover, which pictured three sets of eyes. Inside, Stout described personality and behavioral traits that reminded me of my father, his games of psychological dominance and control. She stated her research, that 4 percent of people are sociopaths: They have an absence of a conscience; they feel no guilt, empathy, shame, or remorse. The question Stout was asked most by her clients was, "How can I tell whom to trust?"

Dr. Ross understood that I had difficulty trusting. He waited and listened. Two years passed before I let him see me cry. When I finally did, I covered my face, leaned over and vomited up my pent-up emotions. Part of me felt I'd lost a battle. Part of me felt afraid of my vulnerability. Part of me felt an unburdening sense of relief.

Quietly, Dr. Ross got up from his chair and placed a box of tissues at my feet.

A little bit at a time, over the course of many months, then years, I shared with Dr. Ross the secret things I'd never told anyone about my father and me.

CHAPTER 6
I'LL MAKE LOVE TO YOU

Dear Future Life Partner,

How many relationships have you had?

I dread this question, which men usually ask me on our very first date. My answer often prompts wide eyes and more questions: Why? What happened? Haven't you wanted to be in a relationship? I offer a stereotypical acceptable response: "I was focused on my career and didn't have time for a love life" or a truer, riskier reply, "I just never met the right guy." But it always feels as if I'm on the defensive, trying to respond to a deeper, unsaid inquiry: What's wrong with you?

People often assume that by a certain age we've had many relationships, but a lack of romantic relationships isn't an equation of our romantic relationship skill or worthiness. I'm telling you this for a reason, of course. Soon, I'll share with you what happened when I dated my first boyfriend.

Here's a bolder question: How do you feel about sex? What I mean is, what's your situational modus operandi? To be candid, I've never felt comfortable with one-night stands and I don't think I ever will. I prefer to have sex only after developing a meaningful connection with my partner. I'm not saying we'd have to wait months, or that once we're a couple a quickie would be off the table. What I am saying is that casual sex isn't for me. I'd never sleep with someone I just met. I'm more into "love making" than "fucking." That's just the way I am.

How do you feel about what I'm saying?

This is hard for me to admit, but for a long time my stance around sex was a source of shame for me—I believed my preferences made me abnormal, unattractive, and unacceptable. But such a viewpoint was rooted in what I'd learned about my value as a partner when I was sexually abused. It wasn't until I'd been through years

of therapy that I came to understand how my shame was tied to the incest I'd suf-
fered, and that my shame wasn't mine—it belonged to my abuser. The more I
healed, the more I realized that we all have preferences and challenges around sex—
shame has no place in this arena—and our sexual status doesn't define our worth.

For a while, painful experiences held me back from taking the risk to love and be
loved. Although it's easier to deny than to admit the depth of a personal impediment
around intimacy, when we have the courage to face the facts of it, we can break the
power it has over us and change our (love) lives.

Love Cat

BEFORE I WAS ready to be with a partner, I learned about companionship another way.

My first long-term relationship was with a cat. I was a thirty-two-year-old college writing professor in the early stages of PTSD recovery, standing inside Mainly Meows, a cat shelter just beyond Somerville, in Cambridge, peering at a huddled runny-nosed sabo-tabby, when a flash of light ricocheted off the shiny metal bars of the animal cages, catching my eye. I looked up to see a tall dark-haired woman in the entranceway. With one arm, she held the door open; with the other, she dropped a small plastic animal carrier to the floor. She exited quickly and then reappeared with a disheveled scratching post, which she flung from her grasp as if it were deadweight.

"Is that it then?" she barked at no one in particular. She did not wait for an answer but turned her back, and, with a brusque hand, slammed the door behind her.

There was a moment of silence, the air filled with some kind of shell-shock, which was broken, finally, by a loud, long meow that leapt up from the floor.

———————

I was never going to have a pet. My father said so. When I was a girl, I begged for a puppy, but the answer was always "no."

"Why?" I asked.

"Because I'm allergic," my father answered.

"A pet is a lot of responsibility," my mother added.

But still, I insisted, I wanted a companion.

"I'll be your dog," my father said.

He got down on all fours. As my mother soaped and rinsed dishes in the kitchen sink, I followed my father into the living room, where I got down on the floor with him and we played a game called "Doggy." Our tongues were hanging out of our mouths, we were panting and sniffing at each other the way dogs do. Suddenly, my father pushed me over. I was on my back. My father laid his body on top of mine. Our eyes met: He had me. I thought I was going to suffocate under his weight. He stuck his tongue in my mouth and laughed like a devil before he let me go.

(I'd avoid dogs for decades until, one day far off in the future, years into my PTSD recovery, Dr. Ross would bring to the office his new puppy, Sherman, a flat-coated retriever who couldn't stay home alone. At first Sherman would jar the hell out of my nervous system with his jumpy puppy behavior, and I'd tell Dr. Ross that if Sherman stayed I'd have to go; the mere sight of his eyes and mouth and tongue made me want to run out the door. But this became an opportunity to overcome my fear and reclaim something my father had taken away from me: my love of dogs. I couldn't foresee that, over time, as we grew to know each other, Sherman would become a comfort to me, grounding me as he fell asleep on top of my feet, his paws gently wrapped around my ankles while he snored; when I became upset, he'd sit up beside me and lean his head into my hands while I rubbed his ears.)

———————

My current landlord didn't allow pets, but when the building's central fire alarm sounded and the tenants poured outside to stand by the curb, several feline faces appeared in the windowsills, staring out at the world.

I lived in a studio, an efficiency unit located on the second floor of a building constructed originally as a hotel in the 1920s. Larger than a typical studio, my apartment included an eat-in kitchen and a small alcove where I could fit a basic writing desk and a couple of storage bins for my clothes. Adjacent to the alcove was a tiny bathroom, where the tub's finish was long gone, and the sink had separate hot and cold faucets. I placed a litter box in the only space remaining: next to the heating pipes, on the wall opposite the power-flush toilet.

My bed took up a third of the studio room. I pushed it up against the far wall so that I faced the front door while I slept, or half-slept, as I did in my

PTSD-driven "high alert" state, waiting for what I thought would be an inevitable, unpreventable break-in. Behind my head was a window and fire escape, and, to my left, two more windows, which overlooked the back of the building. My two jam-packed bookshelves, which I'd bought at Staples and assembled myself, stood against the wall directly across from my bed. My loveseat ran along the periphery of the studio wall and met up with two large stacked corner storage bins, atop which was my small television set with rabbit-ear antennae.

The apartment had one closet, two-feet wide and two-feet deep, located by the front door. I could barely fit my work clothes and winter coat inside it. Two teardrop wall lights did a dim job of illuminating the place.

I was no longer working my panic-attack-inducing job with the verbally abusive boss but was in my fourth year of my first full-time faculty position at a university, an entry-level writing lecturer position. When I told my mother that I was considering adopting, she threw questions at me like rocks: What if the cat got sick, how would I pay the vet bill? I was a poorly paid, low-level professor. I could barely make ends meet. What if I got attached and the cat died? What if my landlord found out and I got evicted? She pointed out the catastrophic things that might happen if I took a step forward.

Clutching an adoption application in my hands, I wavered between two rows of shelved organic canned wet food, kibble, and a variety of carriers, brushes and combs. I wasn't going to go through with it.

Mainly Meows was a small shelter, consisting of only the manager, who was a short athletic woman in her forties, sporting a blonde pixie cut with bangs. Her husband, a dark-haired man in blue jeans and a button-down shirt, appeared as her begrudgingly compliant assistant to whom orders were dispensed in exasperated tones. With the help of one volunteer, a college girl, Mainly Meows set up shop—only three cages displayed at a time—in the window of Animal Ohm, a cramped holistic pet supply store on Massachusetts Avenue, on Saturday afternoons.

The cat's name was Hannah. Her tail tip was broken, her crème-calico coat smelled of garbage, and her ears were plugged with dirt. She flinched whenever a hand went near her. She watched me over the shoulder of the shelter manager who held her. Gazing at her large green eyes, I thought she looked like Betty

Davis, or Katharine Hepburn in *The Philadelphia Story*. I thought she embodied bravery, tenacity, and heart.

I wanted her in my life.

"The story," the shelter manager shook her head as she spoke to her volunteer, whose eyebrows curved upward with intrigue, "is that woman was a friend of the owner, a man whose young daughter was *bored* by the cat." She sighed as if the information was intolerable, her face darkening in disgust. "He gave her to his *friend*, who says she was *annoying* and *needy*."

I winced. I'd heard those emphatic labels directed at me by ex-friends.

The volunteer pulled on her wispy auburn ponytail and scrunched her nose, making crinkle lines on her forehead. "She's stinky," she said.

"Can I pet her a little?" I asked.

"Yes," the shelter manager granted permission, adding, "she's calm now," though Hannah, whose overgrown claws clung to the shelter manager's T-shirt, still seemed quite agitated. I felt nervous, worrying she might bite.

Hannah kept her attention on me, steadfast, as I touched the light brown and beige shades of fur on the top of her head and traced the softness between the translucent apricot flaps of her ears.

"Hi," I said.

Hannah blinked.

My gaze followed the whiteness that led from the middle of her forehead and down her face, where a cluster of brown fur created a moustache-like marking that framed her pink nose and mouth.

The shelter manager spoke to the volunteer in a low and sobered whisper about abuse and neglect, and then pulled Hannah away. "We'll let her chill down here for a bit," she said, bending over to place Hannah in a cage to be pushed in the darkness under a covered table.

As I watched the cage door begin to close, I said, "I'll take her."

————————

Three days later, after Hannah was health-checked by a vet, the Mainly Meows manager brought her to my apartment building, where she inspected my studio for "cat-proof" clearance before allowing Hannah out of the carrier. She took one look at my tan micro-fiber loveseat, which I had covered with a clear plastic shower curtain, and almost denied the adoption.

"The cat is going to go on the couch," the manager murmured, her blonde eyebrows pressing downward. "Maybe this isn't the home for her."

I am certain I seemed like a crazy woman. Looking back, it's a wonder the shelter manager didn't immediately take Hannah and leave the premises. I'd covered the loveseat to protect myself; I didn't want a cat—I didn't want *any*one—to touch my things. I was afraid that Hannah would contaminate me and cause me to die. I didn't have a cat allergy (I'd been tested and cleared); rather, this was a symptom of my fear of intimacy, which I'd only begun to explore in therapy.

But something larger than my fear, perhaps my innate capacity to love and be loved, surged in my chest, pushed against my collarbones and up into my throat: "Yes, it is," I said, and I removed the plastic.

My desire for companionship trumped my phobia.

———

"Don't worry," my mother said resentfully over the phone when I told her about Hannah. "I'll still visit you."

Holding the receiver to my ear, I silently recalled a photograph in one of my childhood albums that pictured my mother in bell-bottom blue jeans placing a stray cat in my arms as we stood beside a wooded area near Lake George, where we were on vacation. I was four years old. I remembered the moment, how the cat approached us, how my mother picked her up, encouraged my interest in this animal, fed my wish for love.

I didn't understand why my mother was so displeased now. I felt hurt by the way she seemed to be trying to hinder my happiness.

She showered me with negativity: "I don't like cats. What if you have an allergic reaction?" she asked. "What kind of name is 'Hannah'?"

Instead of telling my mother that she was being unhelpful, I tried to assuage her worries by telling her I thought adopting a cat would be okay, even though

I wasn't sure myself if that would ultimately be true. I'd grown up with and had adopted my mother's fears. My mother's reaction to my decisions had always been a barometer to which I turned to measure the soundness of my judgment. I didn't want to think that her response was motivated by anything but her love for me; I wanted to believe her comments were merely caused by her need to be overprotective—and yet I ignored how there were crucial times in my past when my mother hadn't been protective at all when it was actually necessary.

Our first night together, Hannah cried. I got out of bed and moved through the darkness, my eyes wide and searching, my ears following the persistent calls, until, with my hand, I found her body on the floor.

I stroked her as soothingly as I could. "It's okay," I said. "It's okay."

Hannah trotted over to her kitty bed, which I'd placed atop a storage bin in the corner of the alcove. She curled herself into a circle, turned her body over and over, and kneaded the puffy fabric. I went to her, and stroked her in the kitty bed. I thought about bringing her into my bed with me, but, as much as I wanted to cuddle, I couldn't bring myself to do it: The idea was overwhelming, too evocative of the trauma of my past that I'd only just started to face.

One night, Hannah decided she was going to join me. She found an opening in the sheets at the foot of my mattress and quickly tunneled up toward me. The quick pounce of a body on my legs sent terror through me like an electric shock. I awoke kicking and screaming *No no no no no!* as if a rapist had come to my bed. Fight or flight: My mind began to spin with the fear and rage of a cornered animal. *Why are you doing this to me?* I yelled out in the darkness, my hands pushing Hannah away. She leapt from my bed and ran.

My limbs shook as I got out of bed. I didn't yet have enough of a handle on my PTSD symptoms to comprehend my visceral feeling of pumping adrenaline as a signal that I was reacting to something from my past trauma and not the present event. All I could think was I had to stop my assailant from coming back to harm me.

I shut Hannah in the bathroom with her food and water bowls so that I could sleep without worrying about being "attacked," and then got back into bed.

After a few minutes, Hannah began to meow with echoing melancholy, louder and louder. A memory flashed in my mind:

When I was four and five years old, my mother often shut me in the bathroom because I refused to poop. She told me I had to sit on the toilet until I went. I cried, calling "Mommy! Mommy!" until she came to the door. "Yes?" she said, as if she expected me to say I had pooped, but I hadn't. I said in between sniffles, "I think I have a cold!" I wanted her to open the door and sit with me. I wanted her to hold my hand. Something was wrong, things were happening to my body, but I didn't have the words to articulate to my mother, or to myself, what those things were. All I knew was I felt mad and sad and scared. My mother answered gently, "You don't have a cold, you're just crying." And then she walked away.

Hannah cried mournful wails from inside the bathroom, increasing in volume. I was afraid she'd wake the neighbors and get me in trouble. Flinging off the covers, I left my bed and opened the bathroom door where I saw Hannah perched atop the toilet seat, her head bowed: She was me at five, sitting there so sad, a hurt and helpless part of myself I thought I couldn't bear to see.

Hannah ran then from the bathroom, and around and around the apartment, jumping on the bed, the loveseat, running across the floor. It was impossible to contain her.

"Why are you doing this to me?" I cried. "I love *you*, why don't you love me back?" I heard how strange my questions sounded, how they didn't match the circumstances. Still, I wept as if my cat should answer me.

Finally, I chased her into a corner and hissed at her so fiercely that her fur flattened with her recoil. I hated myself for what I was doing, thinking, feeling. She was just a cat, but in my triggered state she was my tormentor. I felt ashamed of myself. I thought someone should take her away or arrest me. I didn't deserve her. I didn't deserve love or companionship. I buried my face in my hands, fell into a heap on the floor, and sobbed.

After a long while, I felt a tail reach across my shoulder and brush against my back.

Some days, Hannah told me the story of her past through her body language: When she heard loud voices or heavy footsteps her face became drawn, her ears flapped back, and her body shrank low; if I brought a date home, she gave him a look of terror before she bolted and hid behind the bathroom door; she ate from her food bowl with her body against the wall and dodged off if I approached; she only let me pet her if my hand came from the side. If my hand came toward her face directly, she jumped as if to avoid a blow.

Sometimes, when I touched her, she froze for a moment before she eased, then turned her body around and around in her kitty bed, kneading as I stroked her. She caught the soft fabric in her claws and tugged it toward herself as if it were a security blanket.

Sometimes she entered a kind of spell, as if the past were taking hold like a riptide, pulling her away. Such an episode was usually preceded by loud noises or footsteps. She huddled in a "duck-and-cover" position behind the bathroom door, in the corner of the studio alcove, or beside or under my bed, her body lying low to the floor, as if she were trying to disappear into it. I watched her eyes glaze over as if a screen had been lowered, as if some kind of vision were coming down upon her, playing out within her mind's eye, lasting for minutes, sometimes hours.

"Hannah," I called to her softly, but she wouldn't look at me. I tried to catch her gaze. I called to her a little more firmly, "Hannah." But she'd closed her ears, as if to close up herself. She stared as if she were in a trance, gone to another time and place. I wondered if her past was flashing before her in the way mine often did.

"Hannah," I called to her once more, placing my palm lightly on her back. She moved out from under me, her attention scattering, her eyes dashing across the floor as if it were projecting a horror film. "Hannah, it's okay."

I waited with her until, finally, she emerged as if from a cocoon. Her body eased. She stood, sniffed my hand, pressed her cheek to my arm, lifted her nose up to my face, and looked into my eyes, where what had gripped her and wound her so tightly lost its hold.

Hannah and I triggered each other at the same time we were catalysts for each other's healing.

———

My PTSD diagnosis came a little less than a year after I began therapy with Dr. Ross.

My father, who'd recovered from the metastatic lung cancer, called me on my twenty-ninth birthday to tell me that Donna had been diagnosed with uterine cancer.

"She has pain when we have sex," he cried.

It was as if he poured lava over my body: my head then shoulders then torso then legs turned too hot, then numb. I barely breathed. I told my father I was sorry, rushed him off the phone, and tried to forget what I'd heard, the words "pain" and "sex." *You're being too sensitive*, I silently chastised myself. *Stop it.*

Suddenly, memories of the sexual abuse of my childhood exited the vault where I'd locked them inside myself, where I'd stored the truth for decades. Over the next several days and weeks, it was as if my mind were a roll of masking tape, my consciousness unsticking layer after layer, dispensing my past, piece after piece. Unfurling the whole story would take years.

———

A few months after my revelation, I sat alone with my mother in her condo living room (she'd sold our Long Island home a few years after the divorce, and moved to a community near Westchester), the framed photos of my brother and me as children watching from the mantel like witnesses as I took the lid off the silence of our family.

"There's something I want to tell you," I began. "It's very difficult to share."

"You can tell me anything," my mother said.

I worried she'd become angry with me, or so bereft that I'd be unable to console her. But I felt I could no longer live my life pretending that what happened hadn't occurred. The effects of doing so were too pervasive and debilitating. I wanted to heal so that I could have a chance at life. Speaking the truth was a first step.

I held my breath. "When I was growing up," I began, "Dad sexually abused me."

My mother's eyes widened but her voice remained unemotional. "When did this happen?" she asked. "Where was I?"

I kept my voice even, matching my mother's tone so as to soothe her. I didn't want to overwhelm her with too many details at once. "There were many instances over many years," I said. "Sometimes you were reading in the living room, or you were asleep in bed."

My mother's eyes became glassy and fixed. "I think you were too sensitive," she said. "Some other little girl would've liked it."

My breath left me as if I'd been sucker punched. She mustn't have spoken what she had—my mother wouldn't, couldn't—I thought. At the same time, I thought about whether she was right.

"Why are you telling me this?" she asked, her voice falling flat.

Hopelessness pulled at my ribs. "I thought it might bring us closer," I said. I'd felt we were so distant.

"Why didn't you tell me when it happened?" she asked, her voice tinged with accusation. Her eyes wouldn't meet mine.

I felt as if I was testifying in court; my mother had called me to the stand, and I didn't have an answer. I was at fault.

"I don't know," I said. As a girl, I couldn't bear the reality. Our family didn't allow for the acknowledgment of such a truth, though we all lived with it. I didn't think I could explain this to my mother. I had trouble comprehending it myself.

My mother kept her eyes cast downward and let out a half-sigh. Then she pursed her lips. "When your father and I were seeing Dr. Tetley," she said, "he said 'the children show signs of abuse.'"

I hadn't heard him say such a thing when I was there.

"What did he mean?" I asked, suddenly feeling validated, hoping that my mother might now become a source of support for me. She could help me heal.

"I don't know." She waved her hand in the air as if to brush it aside. "I didn't ask."

"What do you mean you didn't ask?" How could my mother, or a trained therapist, let something like that go?

"He said it in passing on our way out," she added.

"He wasn't a very good therapist," I said. "He should've done something."

"No," my mother disagreed. "He was a very good therapist. Seeing him, I got out all my anger about my father." My mother's father had died of Hodgkin's disease when she was twenty and away at college. Her family had kept the graveness of his illness from her, and, as a result, she'd never had the chance to say goodbye.

For a moment, I stared into my lap, at my clenched hands.

"Do you think he abused your brother?" my mother asked.

"I don't know," I said, feeling irritation rise in my chest. I was angry at the way my mother had focused on my brother when we were kids to the point of overlooking the devastating things that were happening to me. She was still doing it. "You'll have to ask *him*. I'm talking about *me* here." I felt selfish saying the words, but I couldn't stop myself.

My mother's eyes appeared sober. "The most important thing in my life," she said, "was to raise my children. If your father sexually abused you, then my whole life's work is a failure."

Then she stood and left the room.

I followed her to her washer and dryer, where she began to sort her laundry. The space between us was filled with a static hush, until, as my mother focused her gaze inside the mouth of the washing machine, transferring her clothes to the dryer, she spoke: "I remember," she began very quietly, "when I caught you masturbating in your bed."

"What?" I asked. My breath grew shallow.

"You don't remember?" she said, her fingers grasping at her wet underwear. "You were seven or eight."

I knew I'd masturbated as a teen, but I didn't recall doing so as a younger child. My mind began to spin. "I don't remember that at all," I said. I thought that if I'd done it I'd remember it—but then I reminded myself of the concept of dissociation. It felt strange to hear my mother tell me something I had no memory of, but I believed her. I was compiling a more complete picture of my past. I asked, "What was I doing?"

"I don't know," my mother sighed, her eyes remaining on the task at hand: She reached into the washer basin, unfolded a bunched-up handful of clothing, then tossed it into the dryer with the flick of her wrist. "It was after you had been put to bed. I walked by your room." Her voice escalated: "You had the comforter between your legs and you were riding it!"

"What did you do when you saw?" I asked.

"I asked you what you were doing," she said. "I asked you if you liked it."

"What did I say?" I pressed. Why did I have to ask these questions? Why didn't she just offer up the entire story, tell me everything she knew? What was she afraid of? What was she withholding?

"Nothing," she said, as her hands rummaged through her cotton nightgown, which she then buried in the dryer. Her eyes remained fixed on the laundry. "You just laughed."

I crossed my arms, feeling a chill. What my mother described sounded like a trauma-induced trance state. "I didn't say anything?"

"No," she said, her tone pushing back. "You don't remember?" For a brief moment she looked at me. "I told you to stop but you kept doing it." Then she looked back at the underwear, which she untwisted and threw into the dryer. "So I got you a book to read about it. For all I knew you were going to get your period early or something. Sometimes girls feel ashamed about that kind of thing."

As I watched my mother clean the lint trap, I wondered if she believed I should have felt ashamed then, and if I should feel ashamed now in the presence of this memory. This bothered me, but what upset me more was that something so bad had happened to me that it had caused me to block out my memory of an incident my mother had clearly witnessed. Then she reminded me of when I began to leave my room in the night and sleepwalk. "Maybe you were trying to escape," she said, throwing up her hands.

"Did you tell anyone about it?" I asked about the masturbation.

"No," she fumbled with more laundry. "Like who?"

"I don't know," I said. "What about Aunt Nikki? If you thought it was abnormal or something, maybe you'd check it out with your friends who had girls? Or the pediatrician."

"When we saw the pediatrician," my mother said, "I had too many things to discuss with him regarding Russell's problems adjusting in school. I didn't have time for anything else."

"Did you tell Dad?" I asked.

"Probably," she said. "We talked about things."

My mother's words were becoming slippery, noncommittal.

"What did he think about it?" I asked.

"He thought it was funny. We joked about it."

I sensed she was tired of talking, but I felt as if there was more she wasn't revealing.

"When I was really little," I reminded her, "I had trouble going to the bathroom."

My mother interrupted. "I fixed that," she said quickly, her eyes darting. "I took care of that."

"Sometimes I told you I was sore between my legs," I added.

"Yes," she said, tossing a fabric softener sheet into the dryer, then closing the lid. "Children have all sorts of issues. It doesn't mean they're being sexually abused. I would've known if something was going on. I was your mother."

She began to place another load of laundry into the washer, this time colored clothes—pants, shirts, socks—which she methodically arranged. She couldn't just let it all tumble out of the basket and into the washer bin. She could never allow the color clothes, however light, to mix with the underwear, unless they were as white as the panties, which she bleached, though they had irremovable stains in the crotches.

"Did you ever see anything in my underwear?" I asked.

"No," she said, not pausing to first think back, as if she was afraid to remember. "Why are you asking me that?"

"There are some gaps in my memory," I said, "and if you remember anything, anything at all, it could really be of help to me if you tell me."

"I don't remember anything other than what I told you," she said, her fore-finger pressing the "colors" button.

She was done.

I backed off, took a step away.

Then my mother wiped her hands and turned toward me, her eyes suddenly searching mine. Her face crumpled, and she began to sob. "I know it happened, there were signs!" she said, flinging her body upon mine as if she were letting go of herself. I stepped back into her bedroom doorway in a kind of stupor. She felt smaller in my arms than I remembered, her body delicate. "I wish it had happened to me instead!"

I held my mother as I would a child.

"No," I said, as a strange sense of death came over me. I heard my voice outside myself, without emotion. "It's okay," I said. The more my mother's body shook in mine, the more my voice grew quieter.

I remembered when things got really tense between my parents when I was in high school and I kept my mother company until she fell asleep on a cot she bought for what she called "the fourth bedroom," a tiny spare room that she'd converted a few years earlier from a playroom into an office space where she completed her copyediting assignments and where she wrote poetry and essays. *I'm sixteen years old*, I'd think on a Saturday night while the other kids I knew were out, *but I can't leave my mother*. I worried when I went to the prom, when I left home for college, *who'll take care of her now?* She told me she'd be okay, that she could take care of herself. "Don't worry about me," she always said with a smile, but there was something about the pitch of her voice, the dash of her eyes, the movement of her lips, the way her shoulders turned inward, that made me believe that underneath it all she wasn't telling me what she really thought and felt.

Now, the way my mother alternated between denial and acknowledgment both confused and troubled me.

"If there's anything I can do—" she started but then stopped, as if she were unwilling or unable.

"The way you can help me now," I said, "is to answer any questions I might have, tell me anything you might remember."

She grew very still. In that moment, I understood that my mother wasn't going to help me. I took her arms in my hands and lifted her body away from my own. "I need you to take care of yourself," I said. My mother looked up at me with a tear-stained face, with watery pads beneath her eyes. I continued, "I need for you to take care of your feelings about this with a friend or a professional, so that I can cope with this myself."

She nodded in obedience, said "okay," as she gulped another sob, and then, with what was laced with a tinge of bitterness, "I know you hate it when I cry."

I'd never told her that. I wondered who, in her past, had.

———

In the weeks that followed, my mother decided to see a social worker once a month, a woman who ran a local battered women's shelter, "so that I can understand you," she said to me. She said she didn't need therapy for herself.

After her first appointment, she called. "I made a mistake in the way I first reacted," she said. "I should have been supportive. Now I can help you heal, if you'll let me."

I wanted to let her.

For the next several months, each time we talked on the phone she broached the subject by saying, "How's the therapy going?" When I said I was struggling with flashbacks and painful emotions she interrupted and said, "I can't hear the details." I didn't know how to tell her what was going on without being specific. "You can be general," she said. But I couldn't be general enough for her comfort level, so I stopped discussing it except to say in response to her question about "the therapy" that I was going to my sessions. Then she claimed I was refusing to let her in: "You refuse my offer to help you heal," she said, speaking clinically. She peppered our conversations with the language of therapy, as I sometimes did. "You're punishing me for the past," she said, "by withdrawing yourself and withholding information."

"You say you can't hear certain information," I said.

"I need to be able to function," she said. If she heard particular details, she wouldn't be able to get out of bed in the morning, do her laundry, go to work, or live her life.

"That means certain topics will be off limits from our conversations," I said. "Our relationship will be limited."

"Yes," she said. "I wasn't there for you then, but now I can be, if you'll let me."

I seriously wondered if there was something wrong with me because I didn't follow my mother's line of logic.

"It's time for you to move on," she said.

It wasn't as simple as that.

———

In my sessions with Dr. Ross, I began to examine the ways my past trauma informed my present-day life. I started to become cognizant of just how Hannah triggered me, and the ways I placed myself in the role of a victim with abusive bosses and "friends" who used me. I went on dates with often jerky and narcissistic men I met online, though I thought I'd made careful selections on the dating site: He had a steady job, he didn't look like my father, and he didn't mention his urgent need for sex in his profile. I didn't consider any man more than five years older than me, or any man who owned a dog, though a man with a cat was allowed. I blocked from my account men who were old enough to be my father and who sent me messages about my physical beauty, detailing what they wanted to do to my body, making my stomach turn.

Before my dates, I spent hours in the bathroom, sitting on the toilet crying, with my stomach in knots. Hannah sat a few feet away and watched quietly, almost motionless, as if she were taking in my unspoken thoughts, absorbing them from me like a bandage on an oozing wound. Why did I put myself through such torture? I wanted to have a boyfriend, a husband, and a family. I wanted to have a life. I wanted to be normal. Sitting in Starbucks one morning I overheard two women in their mid-twenties discussing their upcoming weddings: "Can you imagine not being married by the time you're thirty?" They sighed with relief. I left the Starbucks in tears.

When it was time to leave for a date, my body shook and folded into a pile in the middle of the studio floor. There, Hannah circled me, every so often nudging the side of my arm with her nose and the top of her head. I looked in her eyes and let her comfort me like a mother consoling her girl.

I got up from the floor and made my way out into the world, knowing Hannah would be there for me when I returned. When I opened my apartment door, she greeted me with several enthusiastic meows, as if to say, "Tell me details!" as she leapt to her cat bed in anticipation. I knelt beside her, taking in the calmness of her purring, the warm vibration in my hand, until the shakiness in the backs of my thighs, and my mind, subsided.

One evening, my date arrived late at the Newbury Street bar he selected, carrying his gym bag, informing me he would've been there sooner had he not stopped off at a store down the block to buy a gold watch. Over drinks, he proceeded to fill the air with a story about a woman he once took out, how she got very drunk, how he took her home, how *she* seduced *him*, he said, how men find that very flattering, and how he spent the night with her. I wondered if that was the scenario he planned for me. I left quickly, feeling frightened.

I wished to be lucky enough to find you: someone decent, nice. But I wasn't yet ready. In the early stages of PTSD recovery, I was unconsciously trying to work out what I never could with my father. What is the definition of insanity? Doing the same thing over and over again but expecting a different outcome.

I went on date after date, trying to find "a better fit": I saw Geoff, the guy with the black leather jacket and Mercury LeSable, whom I kissed after our second date while standing at the foot of my bed and who went shopping with his mother every weekend thereafter, and therefore was too busy to see me; I met Vincent, a man I suspected was high when he showed up at our meeting place, Starbucks, sweating profusely, his eyes bugged out and jittery, and who claimed his cousins were the Coen brothers and who wanted to just "go for a walk and be alone," at which point I promptly ended our date; I went out with Lee, who took me to dinner and then took a long break outside to talk on the phone with some other woman.

Although I wasn't finding "a better fit," I found that the more dates I went on the more I began to parse out my past from the present moment. I started to hear my inner voice and trust my gut.

———————

The more I reckoned with my history, the more I came into conflict with my mother.

When my mother visited, we fought in front of Hannah, who sat in her kitty bed, her tail waving its crooked end, which pointed inward, as if to the soul-breaking events of her past.

"I don't understand," my mother said, her voice rising, "where your anger toward me comes from. I didn't *do* anything. Your father was the one—" She suspended the end of her thought.

"You were sitting in the next room when it happened," I said. "You didn't stop him."

"I didn't know!" she said. "You never said anything."

I had no response.

"As I've said before, I'm sorry it happened," she said.

"Anyone can say they're sorry 'it' happened," I said. "You never say you're sorry for your part."

"My part?" she said. "I didn't abuse you. If I had known what was going on I would've done something, but you never said anything, no one from outside ever said 'something looks wrong between Tracy and her father,' no one ever told me—" She stopped mid-sentence, crossed her arms, and held her elbows with her fingertips.

If she had known? I thought to myself. She'd previously said she had.

I studied my mother: Her hair looked brassy-brittle under my halogen lamp-light. Her blue eyes appeared swollen behind her glasses.

She spoke as if she were in a trance: "I had panic attacks when your brother was five. I had trouble swallowing meals." She said it in monotone, as if she were reading a grocery list. "I had trouble breathing while driving the car with you two in it. I'm sure as kids you and Russell picked up on that vulnerability. I thought I was crazy, but really it was that your father was controlling my mind, telling me that my perceptions were wrong. He manipulated me."

For the first time, I saw my mother's frailty. When exactly had she become this way? I didn't want to see that this had always been the way she was. Many times, in my early teens and twenties, if I expressed some minor discontent with something my mother had said or done, she became annoyed: "You and your brother expect me to be perfect," she often said. "You don't allow me to be human." I didn't expect my mother to be infallible. In fact, I felt she was the one who always needed me to be. But in truth, for my whole life I'd idealized her, because I couldn't bear to face the fact that she'd failed me. Now, seeing her in this light, I felt shock and frustration, and grief.

"I'm sorry for all that you went through," I said. "But you were my mother."

"How could you be raped," she said, "and not make a noise?"

"Are you saying you don't believe me?" I asked.

"No," she said. "I already said I believe you."

I wasn't sure I believed her: Why was there this debate?

"Why," she continued, "did I not hear a scuffle?"

"I left my body," I said, grasping at therapy jargon to more easily explain a coping mechanism I didn't think my mother would accept.

"Rape is violent," she said. "I would've heard it happening. How could I not know, when I was sitting ten feet away in the other room?"

"Maybe you weren't capable," I said. "Maybe you were so traumatized by Dad that you were blind to it."

"Well then," she said, "if I wasn't capable, how can you hold me accountable and be angry with me?"

"Because," I said, feeling outrage at what I saw as her attempt to exonerate herself, "I was a helpless child and you were my parent! What did you think he was doing in my room for so long?"

"I thought he was reading you a bedtime story!"

"Dad *never* read to me! Only *you* did!"

Hannah leapt from her cat bed to the middle of the floor, between my mother and me. She sat there contemplatively.

When I was a girl, every night my mother read to me. She bathed me. Every day, she combed my hair, dressed and undressed me. She taught me how to tie my shoes and zip my coat. She gave me hugs and kisses. But I always sensed there was a part of her that was turned the other way, distracted, her attention centered around helping Russell.

When Russell was in fourth grade and I was in kindergarten, my mother told me that my teacher, Mrs. Sierra, said, "Tracy is such a substantial child."

"What's 'substantial' mean?" I asked.

"It means you can take care of yourself," my mother said with pride.

In kindergarten, I also learned the meaning of the word "embarrassed" when my mother wrote a letter to Mrs. Sierra the day after I had an accident in the classroom, leaking a pool of my urine onto the floor. My mother explained to Mrs. Sierra that I was "embarrassed" for what had happened. She said the problem was that I feared the power flush toilet, which is what I'd told her, but what I really feared was anyone knowing that I had to go to the bathroom, that I had an urge "down there." I had to hide that, above all else. I let Mrs. Sierra believe that what my mother said was true, because I believed my mother always told the truth, so I thought it must be the real truth, but it really wasn't. I couldn't express the real truth, even to myself. I could only stare at the floor as Mrs. Sierra put her arm around me and said it was okay. Only I knew it wasn't.

All those years, my mother made it sound as if I didn't need her. But I did need her, and as I grew up I grew resentful that she chose my brother over me, time and time again, that she deemed him more worthy, more important of her attention and care. It would be decades before I'd look back and see the truth: It wasn't about choosing my brother over me—it was about doing whatever she could to psychologically get herself as far away from my father's grasp as possible, and that included distancing herself from anything associated with him, which in this case was me.

My mother's voice broke through my thoughts, brought me back to the present, in my studio apartment. "I read a story in the *New York Times*," she said, "about a little girl who was raped by her father on the Long Island Rail Road. He put her on his lap and did his thing. She didn't make a sound. A woman across the aisle saw the whole thing and reported it to the conductor and the police met them at the next stop and arrested the man." Then she turned to me and threw up her hands: "What if I *had* known, what would've happened to our family? What would've happened if I'd entered your bedroom in the middle of it all? What would've happened then?"

I ran my hand across Hannah's back. She tapped her tail on my forearm.

"Well," I finally let out what, for a long time, I'd wished had happened, "hopefully you would've called the police and they would've put Dad in jail."

I'd wanted my mother to save me.

"No," my mother said, shaking her head. "No, that would not have happened, because your father would've made up a story about how it wasn't what I thought I saw and I would've been convinced by him."

Her words hit me like a train. Even if she'd seen it happening, my own mother wouldn't have tried to help me. She wouldn't have believed me, or her own eyes. She would've believed my father. He had all the power.

That was how it went on for all those years.

In this moment, I finally understood the depths to which my mother had also been abused by my father.

"I'm sorry you were so traumatized by Dad," I said. "But you were my mother."

"I trusted your father," she said. "He was my husband. That's what women were told to do in those days."

"I was a powerless child," I said.

My mother's eyes moved back and forth across the floor as if she were watching a memory play out. "I was powerless, too," she said.

I decided then that it was time for my mother to go. Leading her to the door, I hugged her goodbye for the night. We exchanged "I love yous" as we always did, and then she was gone. After I put the chain lock in its place, I went into the bathroom and sat on the toilet, my elbows on my thighs and my chin on my fists. I opened my hands and bowed my face into them, and I started to weep. Hannah walked over and sat on the floor by my feet. I let one arm dangle down, my fingertips lightly stroking the fur on her back. Every once in a while, she turned her head and I could feel her whiskers and nose wiping the tears where they had dripped on the back on my hand.

My mother kept insisting *I'm there for you*. When I questioned the consistency of her words and actions she insisted, *I'm the same person I've always been, nothing's changed!* And I had to admit to myself, she was right.

I was the one who was changing.

In the process of confronting the truth of my childhood and its effects on my adult life, I was dismantling the myth of love along with the myth of my mother, the able mother I'd wanted and needed to take care of me: the mother who read to me, who sat and talked with me, the mother who knew everything about me, who knew what to do in every situation, who encountered no problem too large to resolve, who was always in charge and unafraid, who protected me—the mother who'd let nothing and no one get in her way.

Knowledge, she always told me, was *power*.

I was coming to know my mother more fully, this woman who loved me, but who, out of fear, refused to acknowledge, to see, how she'd closed her eyes as if to die and turned away from me. My mother believed it was necessary to forget the truth in order to live. In my thirties, I came to understand that this way of living was, in actuality, a way of dying.

As an adult, as reality came into focus, I felt pulled in opposite directions. I understood I had two choices: to stay asleep, like my mother, to preserve the illusion of a healthy mother-daughter relationship; or to awaken from my denial and truly view a woman who'd been marked by her experience of marital abuse. Only in doing so could I fully separate myself from the past and hope to live a different life, not as a victim, not even as a survivor, but as a whole person, someone who could thrive.

My mother had placed me in a thorny position: I had to choose between denial and truth, her or myself. I couldn't have both. And I knew, if I was still loyally tied to my mother, there was no way I'd ever be free to give myself fully to a partner, to love, to life.

First Boyfriend

WE MET ON eHarmony when I was thirty-three.

Mitch was thirty-five, tall and thin with glasses, and more than balding. I was letting go of my trauma-informed grip on appearances.

At the end of our first date, he walked me to my apartment building and kissed me at the curb, missing my mouth on his first attempt, which made him blush and made me giggle.

"Is he Jewish?" my mother asked over the phone during one of our twice-weekly hour-long chats, which she insisted we schedule in advance, in perpetuity.

"No," I said. I was working in therapy to discard certain beliefs that were limiting my dating life. I was learning to see beyond my mother's prejudices.

"Oh," my mother responded.

I heard her disapproval, and it bothered me. My life was finally beginning to grow in ways I'd hoped, and I wanted her support, as if it were a source of strength I didn't already have within myself and which part of me believed I needed in order to successfully take my next steps into the world.

I'd recently secured a new teaching position. Money was still tight, but I had a tiny bit more to work with and decided to move out of my studio apartment and into a one-bedroom below-market-rate unit on the top floor of a house owned by an old Boston Italian family: Walter, a ninety-seven-year-old father of three, lived on the first floor. His seventy-three-year-old daughter, Margaret, lived below me, on the second floor.

My mother tried to dissuade me from making the upgrade: "What if you run out of money and can't pay your rent?" she asked.

I moved, despite my mother.

———————

As soon as we arrived in our new home with its airy rooms and windows, Hannah began to carry herself differently. She walked taller. She ate more. Her underweight body filled out. So did mine. Together, we grew healthier.

After a therapy session, I sat in the living room on my loveseat with Hannah curled up beside me. I placed my palm where I could feel her body rise and fall as she took in life and let it go. Closing my eyes, I focused on the vibration of her spirit, the feeling of her calm contentedness, her lovingness, like Braille on my hand. She kneaded the backrest and purred, her breath steady and full. Every once in a while, she lifted her nose to blot my tear-drenched knuckles and slid the side of her cheek up my arm.

Then she sped away as if beckoning me to chase her. With abandon, she dashed down the steep staircase that led to the apartment door and waited for me at the bottom. I held on to the railing and followed, feeling beneath my feet the rough grass-green carpet that rolled down the steps like a tongue. When I was almost halfway to the bottom, Hannah emitted chirpy giggle noises and, like a bullet, shot past me up the stairs, tagging my leg with her tail—*you're it!*—opening up feelings within me that I hadn't felt in decades, parts of my spirit I thought I'd lost during the abuse: affection, playfulness, love. Laughter came loose in my throat.

Joy fluttered in my chest.

———————

Each day, I entered the house through the back door, which opened to the foot of a winding staircase with thin maroon-colored grooved grip pads. I passed the first-floor unit's doorway where Walter appeared like Casper the Friendly Ghost, grinning from his chair at the kitchen table, his large face pale and oblong, his white eyebrows raised. Seated beside him, playing cards, was Dean, his sixty-eight-year-old son, who lived twenty minutes away with his kind wife, Dory. Although he didn't live on the premises, Dean acted as my landlord, mowing the lawn, weeding the garden, and repairing what was broken. Dean was a gentle and congenial man, but Hannah pooped on the floor to display her distress whenever he was in our unit for more than a few minutes.

On Sundays, Margaret's grown children and grandchildren congregated for a family supper, filling the house with laughter and loudness. Ascending the staircase, I breathed in the steamy air of pasta and Italian meatballs, or a whole chicken or a roast. As I put my key in my door lock, Margaret opened her back-kitchen door and passed me a full dinner plate, and a piece of cake for dessert.

Hannah announced her presence then with an elongated meow from the other side of my apartment door. Instantly, Margaret's tuxedo cat, King Tut, appeared, sporting his black shiny coat and white paws, pushing his face between Margaret's leg and the edge of the half-closed door, as if his girlfriend was calling.

"Git—back—in—there," Margaret ordered. "He rules his people, not the other way around."

King Tut backed off for a moment but then returned as if Hannah's voice was irresistible. Margaret clucked her tongue and looked down at the cat's midnight face.

"When Keith brought him home," Margaret said, referring to her live-in boyfriend, "he was just a tiny kitten. So tiny!" Then her voice darkened, and she frowned. "I had the option of getting a different kitten, one that had been abused, but I didn't want one who had something happen to it. I don't want to deal with any baggage." She threw her hands down as if to shake out a dust rag. "I said 'I only want a cat with a clean slate.'"

I wondered if she felt the same way about people. I wondered what she'd think about me, if she knew that I was in therapy for PTSD. I never told her why I never let Hannah meet King Tut face-to-face: Irrational as it may sound, I was afraid he might rape her.

Such anxieties, of course, played out in my dating life.

"Moving," Mitch said, drawing upon his expertise as a practicing clinical social worker, "is one of the most stressful life events you can have, aside from divorce and death." He told me he thought I was "unbelievably put-together" for the circumstances.

When he arrived at my apartment, Hannah snubbed her nose at him.

I made out with him on my loveseat. Sitting on his lap, facing him, my knees around his hips, I put my hands on his shoulders and leaned my lips to his, kissing him slowly, sensually. He put his hands around my back. He was a fast kisser, and I wanted to show him how much better slow kissing could be. Truth be told, I didn't want to feel as if I was being mauled.

As we kissed, Mitch shared with me that he'd recently ended an eleven-year relationship. He told me there were some problems in the relationship, which he didn't want to discuss. I didn't press him. I didn't tell him about my (lack of) previous relationships. I told him my parents had gotten divorced when I was a college freshman, and that I'd dealt with it in therapy so that I could have a healthy relationship. I withheld the fact that I had PTSD. I didn't tell him that I'd been sexually abused. I didn't reveal that, before him, I hadn't had a real boyfriend. I wanted him to see me as a woman, not as an inexperienced girl, which was how I saw myself through the veil of my shame. I wanted to maintain the sense that I was "unbelievably put-together."

One evening, after we'd been seeing each other for about a month, we were lying on the loveseat, cuddling. With my ear on Mitch's chest, I could hear his heart beating and the vibration of his voice speaking, and I remembered how I used to do that with my father. Mitch nuzzled the side of his face against mine and brushed aside my hair with his hand. I knew what he wanted then. I looked up at him.

He dove into my mouth as if I was a pool and his tongue was his whole body. His lips were on mine, and his torso moved rhythmically, and I envied the freedom he seemed to feel. I felt paralyzed with my spine pushed to the back of the loveseat. As he thrust his tongue all I could think was *he's having sex with my mouth*, but I didn't want to think so I shoved the thought away as he pulled me in to his body with one hand and moved his other hand up my side, from my waist to my breast and I felt something, *yes,* and then I felt proud *my body works like a normal woman's* and then I was afraid *no, no, no, no, no I don't want to do this, somebody help me.*

Everything was silent, except for Mitch's breathing, which was heavy and deep and long, and I knew he was becoming more and more turned on, and then the terror from my past overtook me and I could no longer push away the scene that was replaying in the back of my mind: I was a girl and this man was my father—*I do but I don't want to be your girlfriend*—I was pulled in by a sexual arousal that possessed me, toxically, I was crossing that point of no return where love becomes tainted and ugly and so do you because it becomes a part of you, this thing that is being forced onto you, into you, what he is doing and what you are doing to you, that causes the destruction of you, everything within you and between you two.

Somewhere down the road, my future self wouldn't become flooded by the past during physical intimacy. But at this point in my journey, I wasn't recovered enough from my trauma to be able to navigate a trigger or flashback while being with a partner. Instead, I tried (unsuccessfully) to compartmentalize it.

I nudged Mitch off me and smiled nervously. "Whew, that was intense," I said, barely breathing as I sat up, trying to keep hidden what was going on inside myself.

For the rest of our time together that evening, I avoided any kind of "make-out" position. Mitch didn't push me to continue, though he didn't inquire as to why I'd stopped either. I was afraid he'd leave me. At the same time, I desperately wanted him to go.

Finally, he went home.

I cleaned wherever he'd been, especially the toilet, drenching the bowl with Lysol. Hannah followed me from room to room, sitting quietly, observing me. I felt sick at the sight of Mitch's bare footprint on the white oval foot rug and wished with intensity to wash it in the hot cycle, to burn out his touch, but the Laundromat was closed at that hour and my sink wasn't sufficient, in my mind, for effective cleansing. I considered throwing the rug in the trash but convinced myself not to, due to the cost of buying another one with my already scant funds. Instead, I vacuumed it.

I knew my reaction was compulsive and obsessive, symptomatic of my PTSD, but still I couldn't stop myself from continuing to clean. Even after I'd gone over the apartment twice, everything still seemed contaminated, especially me. So I got into the shower and turned on the water as hot as I could tolerate and stood there for a long while, scrubbing my arms and legs and chest with a soapy loofah sponge, rinsing and scrubbing, repeating again and again and again, letting the pin-needled stream flow over my body until my skin was pruned, until I could no longer feel anything. Finally, I parted the curtain and stepped out of the tub. I dried myself off with a fresh towel and wrapped a robe around my body, but I still felt dirty.

That night, I dreamed that a man I loved entered my bed. I couldn't see his face, only his naked legs, which were covered with my father's fiery red leg hairs, climbing under the covers to be with me. Sitting up fast, I opened my eyes wide, forcing the nightmare to disintegrate, the image dissolving into the darkness of my surroundings.

———————

Two days later, on a park bench, while we watched the traffic pass, I told Mitch the truth.

"When I was growing up," I stated it as simply and as briefly—cleanly—as I could, "I was sexually abused." I told him I wasn't yet ready to have sex with him. I wanted to, I said, but I needed him to be patient and wait a little while longer. "I'm working very hard in therapy to heal," I explained, "but I need more time."

Mitch's lips parted as if to say something, but then no words came. He sat for a short while, looking down at the pavement, then out at the street, and back down at the pavement again. Then he stood and walked away. Later that night, he sent an email. He wanted to be able to say the right thing, he wrote, but he couldn't.

He ended it: "I'm not up for being the partner of a survivor."

I felt hurt and angry, but not so much at Mitch as at myself. I hated my inadequacy.

For a while after Mitch, I was afraid of a potential boyfriend finding out about my history and breaking up with me over it. I derailed relationships by ending them before they could even begin. For a long time, I didn't take into account something Mitch revealed to me just after he broke up with me: He had his own demons.

I was annoyed with him for ending our relationship by email instead of face to face, after I'd had the balls to be candid in person. So, seconds after I read his email message, I called him. Over the phone, I told him he was a coward. He said he was sorry. I told him I hoped none of his clients were rape survivors, because he obviously had no understanding of trauma. I wasn't a leper, I said. He said he was sorry, again. Then he said, "Look, to be honest, I'm ashamed of my sexuality."

I was taken aback. What did he mean?

He said he wasn't going to go into it. He hung up the phone.

I thought of reasons why a person might feel ashamed of his sexuality. Was Mitch alluding to the fact that he was sexually abused, too? Was he a sex addict? Was he confused about his sexual orientation? Was he just uncomfortable with intimacy? Was it something else?

The truth is, what Mitch meant by his statement doesn't matter. What does matter is the point I failed to recognize at the time: He wasn't willing to earnestly face his issue. I wasn't the only one with a problem. He was hindering his chance at overcoming his own obstacle to having a genuine connection in a relationship. Maybe he didn't break up with me because I was sexually abused, but because I was facing the godawful truth of my past in order to transcend it, an act that scared him more than having sex scared me at the time.

True intimacy, as I learned, requires the courage to bare it all.

Sex Drive

Often, when we least expect it, we receive a kind of clarity that helps us move forward. Sometimes that clarity comes from difficult news, or something unspeakable, as it did for me one day when I was in the car with my mother, when she shared with me a secret about her sex life with my father.

My mother didn't think she could drive by herself. She needed me with her. When I was a teenager, I accompanied her as she drove across the Throgs Neck Bridge on the way to visit somebody in some place I can't remember. All I remember is how everything suddenly became silent as we entered the ramp. As we became attached to land by only a narrow stretch of cement and metal, my mother's body became as still as a tombstone, her back erect, her jaw clamped down, her hands tight and white, frozen around the steering wheel. "Mom –" I started to say but her hand flew up like a wall and I stopped. I understood the unspoken rule: Talking would be catastrophic. The sound of my voice could cause my mother to cause the car to careen off the edge of the bridge. We might plunge to our deaths.

Three years after I told my mother about the abuse, I sat beside her in her car as she drove on a highway in Boston, en route from my apartment to Russell's apartment on the south shore of Massachusetts. Just a few minutes from our destination, my mother spoke, but it was as if she wasn't speaking or breaking the rule: she barely moved her mouth. With her fingers gripping the steering wheel, she stared through the windshield. She didn't take her attention from the road. She didn't look at me. It was as if I was hearing what was voiced only in the privacy of her mind.

"Your father," she began, "he did some things."

One day, when I was nine or ten, my mother found a stash of negatives in the bureau drawer in the master bedroom. Her face got hot. Her heart pulsed like an alarm and sourness flowed through her chest and stomach and then down her legs.

She waited until later that night to place the transparent plastic strips on the gloss-coated surface of their bureau, in front of my father. She said, who are these for? He said, for himself. He'd placed his camera on the dresser and set it on timer. She said, get rid of them, promise, don't you ever take pictures like this again. He said okay and then called her a prude.

They were photographs of them having sex.

When I was twelve, my father took my mother away on a vacation. Her mother was in the hospital, dying of heart disease, and he said he wanted her to *relax*. The flash went off, she heard the film advance, and that's when she knew. She said, I told you, you were never to do that again. He sat up in the hotel bed and shrugged his shoulders: She was being too sensitive again. *Some other woman would like it.*

The next day my father took her to a secluded beach. She went along, she thought it would be nice. But when they got there everybody was naked. She wouldn't get out of the car. My father got angry and called her a prude. That's when she knew, she told herself, that she had to get out of the marriage.

But she didn't. Two years later, she didn't tell Dr. Tetley what had happened. She didn't tell anyone. No one was supposed to find out. It was her secret. It was her fault. She felt ashamed.

She couldn't fathom the idea of her husband turning to her daughter.

"Your father got enough sex from me," my mother said as we exited the highway, "believe me."

She insisted I promise to never tell anyone. I did.

Then she stopped talking, as if she hadn't said a word, as if she'd retreated back into some kind of shell, as if it had all occurred in my imagination, as if none of it had ever happened.

———————

But hell, it happened. And in sharing her story, she validated mine. As I came to know the fuller picture of my father's behavior and his relationship with my mother, I was able to talk back to that unspoken first date question, "What's wrong with you?"

There wasn't anything wrong with me.

Breaking Up Is Hard to Do

WHEN OUR HEARTS have been wounded, it's hard to let go of the fantasy of love. Sometimes we just don't want to believe the cold, hard truth. We might not want to see that our connection with another person isn't love at all. But we'll never find true love until we break up with our toxic ties.

One day, I imagined my future: You were there. We were getting married, about to share a life together. My father was walking me down the aisle with his hand around my waist. All I could think about was how my father was there, with me, holding me, in front of you, my future husband, and all those witnesses. All I could think was that I was living a lie.

The decision to confront my father with the truth bubbled up on a Thursday evening and stuck like a neon sign in my brain. By Saturday afternoon, I'd plotted how it would go, in my mind. On Sunday morning, I scripted the words on a piece of paper, the facts, their life-altering effects, potential responses and rebuttals, words I held in front of me for hours, waiting for the phone to ring, for my father to call, as he always did on Sunday evenings.

I felt like a murderer: I was about to kill pretenses.

In truth, I wasn't prepared. I didn't talk it through first with Dr. Ross, which, in hindsight, I think I should've done. I hadn't thought through the many ways my father might react, how I might lose my inner balance. I was driven by a compulsion to get it done in one fell swoop. I thought it would be okay, because I'd surprise him, I'd catch him off-guard—I'd have the upper hand.

When the phone finally rang, it was like a defibrillator jolting me.

I said, "There's something I want to tell you. I haven't been ready for a long time, but now I'm ready to tell the truth."

"I'm glad," my father responded. "You've been so distant lately."

Did he think so? Had we ever really been close?

I said, "I joined a therapy group for people who were sexually abused as children."

There was silence.

I'd planned in my head that my father would say, "Who sexually abused you?" And my answer would be, "You did, Dad." But he didn't say it.

There was more silence.

Finally, he uttered a question: "What do you mean, sexual abuse?" His voice was calm and even. "I have no clue what you're talking about."

I read my scripted words and wrote down his responses as a means of staying grounded: pen on paper.

"In looking back at certain things that went on between you and me," I said, "I have come to realize there were many behaviors that were not appropriate between a father and a daughter."

He said, "Like what?"

I anticipated his question, but I didn't think it would be so humiliating to speak the answer. I quickly described some of the things we'd done.

He extinguished them, one by one: "You thought that was *passionate*?" he chided. "You liked it, you invited it, so how could there have been anything wrong with it?"

I became a mechanical doll, putting out my pre-recorded answers: "A child does not understand what is inappropriate, a child is not capable of controlling that kind of situation, that is for a parent to do. I just wanted to be close to you. That was the way."

My father laughed and then his voice turned loathsome: "What the fuck is this sexual abuse." It was not a question, but a statement filled with the sound of his hatred for me. "This sounds like something that came from your mother," he said.

"This has nothing to do with Mom," I said, returning to my written words. "This is between you and me. It has caused me deep confusion, pain, anger, and sadness. It has taken away my sense of trust, my sense of self, and my sense of love and protection. If you can't speak to me in a respectful, caring way, then you're going to have to give me space. I love you but I'm going to have to get off the phone now."

Did I really love him?

"*Sweetheart*," he said, "I *always* treat you in a respectful and caring way."

"No, you don't," I said, but I felt myself slipping away from my conviction, beginning to believe him. I was starting to think that perhaps I'd made a terrible mistake.

"I don't know what you're talking about!" he exclaimed. His words picked up speed like an avalanche, syllabic rocks tumbling toward me, on top of me. "I just don't get it! Your interpretation is wrong! If there's anything I've ever done, then I can't tell you how sorry I am that it happened, but I cannot conceive of anything I ever did! It was never sexually oriented! I never made sexual advances on you! You don't know how hurtful it is to hear from a daughter that her father sexually abused her! It's worse than sticking a knife in someone's chest, you might as well just do that!"

This was before the term "gaslight" was a daily societal conversation.

My father sounded as if he fully believed that what he was saying was the truth, and I began to question myself. I continued to write his words down in order to physically separate, to extricate, myself from them, him, to make the intangible tangible, to get his voice out from inside of me. But I felt myself yielding to his tones, losing my sense of boundaries, where my father started, where I began.

I referred to my script once more: "It's easier to blame me than to blame you, isn't it? Do you think I wanted this to be true? I tried to make it untrue. I silenced myself year after year so that I wouldn't hurt you, but meanwhile you continued to hurt me. You didn't think about how your actions would affect me, only about what you needed and wanted at that particular moment. You used me to gratify those needs and wants. You still do in many ways."

Part of me had naively hoped that my father would respond rationally and empathically, that he'd apologize and try to make amends.

"I didn't do it to hurt you," he said. "I only did it to love you." His voice became funereal: "Now I understand a lot of things."

I mistook his tone for remorse. "Like what?"

"Like why you didn't come to the hospital when I had the brain tumor," he said, sounding as if he were about to cry. "You didn't want to be near me. It would've been too painful for you."

"I didn't come because I didn't know until two days after the fact," I said to assuage my guilt. Of course, I hadn't gone then, either. I'd waited two weeks, though I'd called.

There was a pause, and then my father continued, his voice devoid of emotion: "There's a difference between agreement and interpretation. Your sense of truth and reality is different from any truth I would interpret. I didn't do anything you didn't want. I didn't do anything you didn't ask for or like. Maybe I hugged you a little too hard, but I never made sexual advances."

I felt my brain spin the way it had during the abuse. I was becoming disoriented, confused. I was losing ground. I tried to regain my footing: "Why would I spend all this time being in so much pain if what I said happened wasn't true?" I asked.

"To get back at me for the divorce," he said.

"Why would I want to be so unhappy?" I continued. "I wouldn't. Why do I have nightmares, flashbacks, and panic attacks in the middle of the night?"

"I don't know why you have nightmares," he said.

I kept going, trying to fight back with my father's own weapon: logic.

"Why would I want to suffer, by myself? I wouldn't," I said. "Why would I want to go to therapy, spend all this time and money talking about something that I say affected me deeply if it wasn't true? When it comes to the truth, there is no agreeing or disagreeing, the truth just *is*, and if you don't agree, you can do some research on the subject. Your disagreeing doesn't change the truth of what happened."

"Your *interpretation* of what happened," he corrected me.

"So, you're saying that everything I experienced never happened?"

"Yes," he said. "You have the choice whether or not to think as you do or as I do. If you want to enough, you can change your mind."

Then I heard him speaking but I could no longer take in the words. It was as if something switched off in my brain. I ceased to have the ability to process language, to comprehend. This frightened me. I got off the phone and went into the bathroom and cried and cried, until I burst the capillaries under my eyes. When I looked in the mirror, I saw the face of a battered wife.

Like a child, I reflexively went to my mother for comfort, which was a mistake.

"You sound upset," she said over the phone. "What's wrong?"

"I just confronted Dad about the abuse," I said.

"Maybe you want to call me back," she said, "when you're not so upset."

I cut ties with my father by letter, a note I shared first with Dr. Ross. I requested that my father refrain from responding. He replied anyway, with a lengthy missive enumerating many points, a logical argument to convince me that my memories were false and suggesting they might've been implanted by my therapist. He recommended I stop seeing Dr. Ross, citing "false memory syndrome," a term promoted by the False Memory Syndrome Foundation, founded by Pamela and Peter Freyd in the early 1990s, during a time when the news and courts were flooded by child sexual abuse cases. The Freyd's adult daughter had accused Peter of sexually abusing her as a girl, an act Peter denied and pointed to as a confabulation (false memory syndrome was later debunked by scientific research on traumatic memory).

"You can change your perception," my father reiterated, "if you want. If you love me."

He recommended I take medication in order to do so.

He told me I'd ruined his life.

He said that if what he had done to me was sexual abuse then every kid in the country had been sexually abused. He said he'd checked the facts with a few of Donna's friends who were nurses.

"Even I almost believe him," said Dr. Ross, who'd been in practice for twenty years. This wasn't a reflection on my therapist's mental constitution, but a barometer for how convincing abusers can be, not only to their victims but to (psychologically healthy) bystanders.

I didn't think my father would contact me again, but five months later he sent a birthday card. He always sent money on my birthday, a sign of his affection, and I suspected there was some inside. I desperately needed cash, and, even though he'd abused me, part of me still longed for my father's love, as an addict might a drug. I felt an insatiable desire to open the envelope, but I didn't. I brought it to the post office. Holding back sobs, I gave the card to the postman and told him to stamp it "return to sender." I could've written the words myself, but I didn't want my father to be able to touch or hold any hint of me.

The postman looked at the return address, studying it. Then he looked at me. I assumed he understood that this was a card from my father. "You don't want this?" he asked.

It would've been so easy to say *yes, I do.* But I didn't. I wanted the kind of father I couldn't—didn't—have. I was no longer willing to live in accordance with a delusion.

I shook my head, "No."

"Okay," said the postman. He stamped the card and took it away.

————

Over a decade will pass. Free of my father's "mind-fuck" intrusions, I'll do the psychological work necessary to heal. Then one day a Rosh Hashanah card will come. I won't recognize my father's handwriting on the envelope—his hand has become uncharacteristically unsteady (I'll later surmise that he must've found my address on the Internet, since I moved four times since his last communication). I'll open the envelope, read the card and his note, his words, before it hits me in my brain: This is my father, asking that I contact him. This is my abuser, shaming me for my absence. Despite all the therapy, a dissociative episode will come over me.

I'll burn his words in my kitchen sink, and hope that's the end.

But then, on my birthday, another card will arrive. This time, I'll catch myself; I won't open it. I'll bring it to the post office and have them put a block on anything from my father's address.

I'll call Aunt Nikki who, after my PTSD diagnosis, expressed her profound sorrow and her belief in my story. She shared: Once, when she and her husband were on vacation with my parents, my father got into bed with her and tried to grope her, while her husband and my mother were in the same room. He did it so quietly no one knew. She confronted him later, told him that if he ever tried it again she'd tell my mother. She stopped speaking with my father after my parents' divorce.

Now, Aunt Nikki will do the thing my mother never did: She'll intervene. She'll cut through my father's game of perception. She'll be courageous. She'll call him on the phone, tell him that if he ever tries to contact me again she'll go to the police and tell them everything that he did to me when I was a child, and to my mother.

My father will respond by denying the alleged acts, by calling my claims of abuse my "lunacy." But Aunt Nikki will interrupt him. She'll call him by his name. She'll say, "I've known you since you were fourteen. I know what you're capable of. Someday you'll have to answer to God."

My father, for the first time in my life, will have no comeback.

CHAPTER 7

I HAVE A VISION OF LOVE

Dear Future Life Partner,

Okay, I bet that was hard to read. But I think it's important that you know what I've been through, what experiences shaped me on my journey to you. Although there were times when I didn't know which way to turn, I didn't give up—on myself, on life and relationships, or the hope that we'd meet.

I saw each experience as part of a learning curve. In my thirties, while most of my peers had found their life partners, I was relearning the rules of love. I came to realize that love was a healer, not an abuser. Love accompanied my acceptance of the truth, as opposed to my denial of it—of my past and present, of myself, of others, of what was working, of what wasn't—and shined a light that guided me through debilitating darkness.

When I cut ties with my father, physically and psychologically, the axis of my world shifted, and my vision of love began to change. I started to see that love wasn't about control but about letting go—of preconceived notions, of stereotypes, of fear, of expectations, of dominance, of submission, of trying to be someone I wasn't, of wishing someone would become someone else, of forcing love where there was none.

Has your outlook on love changed over the years? Has it broadened or sharpened, flourished or diminished over time? Has it become more self-focused or focused on others, your end-all-be-all only thing you live for or a self-fulfilling prophecy of catastrophe, or something, anything, in between?

The more I dated, the more I gained insights about myself and the more I understood it's futile to try to change a potential partner's basic values, especially regarding love and relationships. At the same time, having a different viewpoint doesn't mean one of us is "incorrect," or that we have to change in order to be lovable. Although incompatibility with someone you're with is disappointing, it's best to walk away—doing so is the only way you'll find your match.

These realizations didn't come quickly for me, as you'll see in the next few stories I'm about to share. My learning process was something Dr. Ross described as akin to climbing a spiral staircase: I was traveling upward but at certain twists and turns of life experience I revisited old habits and beliefs; I dealt with them again, but this time with the knowledge I'd previously gained—I wasn't backtracking, I was integrating healthier ways, at a higher level.

For so long in my life, love was a commodity. Love was about pleasing others in order to keep them close. That's how I was raised. I didn't want to accept that that wasn't love, because if that were the truth, then for my whole life I hadn't really been loved. I didn't know what that might say about me, or my future. It was painful to know, to see. But with age and experience, including dealing with a major life crisis, I found a new perspective, one that helped me to feel more satisfied in really knowing myself, which brought me closer to knowing you.

Remember the "Attracting Your Soul Mate" instructor who said we have to be "in receive mode"? Although I disliked her concept at the time, eventually I came to understand her point. Grasping for love, or running after it, wouldn't attract a healthy relationship. I had to develop self-confidence, and the belief that true love would come to me.

There are many different forms of love: love for a partner, love for yourself, love for your parents or children or friends or pets, love for your vocation, love for your community. They're not all the same—each has its own qualities, its own energy—but they're all based upon our connection with each other.

How do you fashion a connection with a potential life partner? How do you "feel out" love with someone you've just met? Does your attachment develop through physical chemistry or an emotional or intellectual connection, or all of the above?

Do you know love when you see it?

Chemistry

"THERE ARE THREE main reasons why people our age are still single," said Jason, a thirty-six-year-old accountant I met on Match.com, as we waited for our dinner at a burger joint in Harvard Square. This was our third date.

I was a week away from turning thirty-five. I'd heard about so many people who met online, fell in love, and eventually got married. I'd gone out with many men from online dating sites in the year-and-a-half after my breakup with Mitch, but Jason was the first guy I saw beyond date number one. He wasn't the usual suspect who messaged, "My number is xxx, do you want to come over," or "Hello darling, you looking for a fuck buddy?" or "Do you like erotica? The written kind?" I thought I had a tattoo on my virtual forehead that read, "Seeks Losers." Jason changed my mind.

Jason was different. He seemed normal. And, I thought, we had chemistry.

———

At the burger joint, all but two of the burgers on the menu were named after famous politicians, Harvard icons, sports players, or other newsy celebrities: the Burger Supreme, which was the plain burger I ordered, and the Viagra Burger, which Jason ordered, because, he said, he liked blue cheese.

The Viagra arrived, its sticky slobbery whiteness dripping, at about the same time Jason began to tell me the first main reason why people our age were still single. To be honest, I didn't hear it, because I was too busy trying to swallow my own meal while watching him eat the Viagra.

"The second reason," he continued, "is that there's baggage from family or a previous relationship that prevents the person from maintaining anything long-term." He chewed. "And the third is that the person had a traumatic thing happen and so they avoid relationships."

"Which one is it for you?" I asked him before he could ask me.

———

My first date with Jason happened at a café on a Sunday afternoon. Jason had sworn off coffee six months earlier. I told him I'd never developed a taste for it. We bonded over hot chocolate and tea for two hours. Usually, I ended dates after forty-five minutes (or, in the case of Vincent, the high guy who said his cousins were the Coen brothers, twenty minutes). But this one drew me in.

He looked me in the eye the whole time, which was a little unexpected as I'd been convinced for days before our date that I was meeting a man who only had one functioning eyeball, or so it seemed from his profile photo. Truthfully, I'd almost called it off, because I didn't think I could trust a man who couldn't look me in the eye (this wasn't a superficial hangup of mine but one rooted in my trauma, my attunement to my father's mood through his eyes, the tone of his gaze upon me). But Jason, who was fit and blond and an inch shorter than I was, had two working brown eyes and, to me, they were hot.

We talked about our jobs, our hobbies, and our lives, how we'd gotten from "there" to "here." Jason told me that when he was eighteen his brother died in a freak accident and it changed things. I told him that when I was eighteen my parents split up, and it changed things. At the end of our date, I told him I wanted to see him again. I surprised myself. Usually, I ran.

———

Jason put down the Viagra. "I was in a serious relationship in college," he began. "It was a very difficult breakup."

"Oh," I said. "I'm sorry."

His face grew melancholic. The woman broke his heart when he was twenty-three. Their lives were going in separate directions, he concluded. She was married now, with kids. He talked about her Facebook status updates and photos. I sensed he hadn't gotten over her.

"So," he said, "what about you?"

On our second date, we went candlepin bowling. When I arrived, I saw Jason sitting in his car, a brand new shiny white compact Prius, across the street from the alley. I walked up to his window and waved. "I was going to sneak up on you," he said as he opened the door.

"Well," I said playfully, "I beat you to it."

Jason beat me in all three games. Every time he got up to bowl, I found myself looking at his butt. But, unlike on our first date, I didn't feel physically attracted to him. I felt as if I was looking at a blank wall, as if something inside me had shut off. I thought that if I stared long enough, I'd feel a sense of attraction again. I worried my lack of feeling was the PTSD rearing its ugly head. I was so concerned about my PTSD ruining my chances for a relationship that I didn't consider that perhaps I simply was not attracted to the guy after all. I clung to the self-critical belief that I *should* be attracted to him, because he was nice, and normal, because I might not ever find the man I really wanted—you. (The belief that I should take what I could get because I'd never find anyone better had cropped up earlier in my dating life and would still take me some years to shake.)

Jason told me more about his family, who lived in Seattle, and then he asked, "How often do you see your parents?"

Oh no, I thought, *here it comes*. Now he'd find out about my father and then he'd find out about the abuse, and then that would be the end of our dating. I assumed he'd respond the same way Mitch had.

"I see my mother once every few months," I said, treading carefully.

"What about your father?" he asked.

"I cut ties with him a few years ago."

Jason looked at me, as if waiting to hear more. I scrutinized his face. I saw intrigue and I saw alarm. I might have been projecting my own fear: I was anticipating his rejection. I wasn't ready to tell him about the incest. I wanted him to first get to know me more, as a person, not as my history. Still, I wanted to be authentic, so I told him the truth, but in a general way.

"My father is a toxic person," I said, "and I made a decision to live a healthier life."

"That's pretty impressive," Jason said. "We can't help what happens to us in our families growing up, but as adults we can live differently."

"Yes," I said. "It's nice to not be defined by our pasts."

———————

Over the next week, Jason called me frequently. On his way to Trader Joe's. On his way home from Trader Joe's. On his way to heating up the dinner he'd bought at Trader Joe's. From our separate apartments, we chatted for hours on the phone. We discussed the layout of our respective tiny kitchens. Jason caught himself laughing when I caught myself saying I had "microwave envy." Then his cousin passed away and he told me I wouldn't hear from him "for a little while." After five days, I started to think he might've lied about the cousin. I thought I might not ever hear from him again but then he called and asked me out for dinner at the burger joint and a movie. He picked me up in the Prius. When I got into the car, I caught a glimpse of his eyes and I thought I wanted to kiss him.

But something held me back.

———————

Now, we were eating burgers and he was holding what was left of his Viagra, waiting for my answer to his question about why I was still single. I'd been ingesting my burger by drowning small amounts of it with my ginger ale, but now I simply put it down. My mouth was too dry. My throat had closed. My stomach, legs, and arms were trembling.

I took a breath and simply said it: "Something traumatic happened to me when I was a kid and a few years ago it caught up with me and I started to deal with it, and I put relationships on hold."

"Oh," he said, "Wow. I mean you don't have to tell me anything you don't want to, but I'm interested in hearing what happened."

I looked him in the eye. "This may be a deal breaker," I said.

There it was: I set myself up for rejection. I gave the guy an out—*This may be a deal breaker.* Why did I say that? In my mind, it was better to hand him permission to break up with me instead of waiting for him to do it of his own volition.

He was looking at me, waiting, with an anticipatory smile on his face.

"When I was growing up," I said, "my father abused me." I skipped over the word "sexual," to denote what type of abuse, because I worried it would be too much for Jason to hear, though I assumed he'd understand what I'd left unspoken. I hadn't yet figured out how to best disclose my past to a potential partner, what made me comfortable, what might make him bolt.

He looked me in the face, responding without a beat: "That's not a deal breaker."

I didn't know if I believed him.

By this time, the burger joint was closing. We left for the theater, where Alfred Hitchcock's *The 39 Steps*, a movie I'd first seen in a film studies class during graduate school, was playing. We sat in the corner of the balcony. Jason bought a Toblerone chocolate bar and broke off pieces every few minutes, placing them in my hand.

After the movie, he drove me home, and he didn't try to kiss me. I wondered if that was out of respect for what I'd told him over the Viagra, or if he simply wasn't interested.

———

Two days later, he called and asked me out again for the following weekend, my birthday. I wanted to go ice-skating at the Frog Pond at Boston Common.

"I can think of no other person," I said, "who'd be more fun to go with."

He said, "I feel the same way."

The next night, he called again.

After an hour and ten minutes of chitchat, he finally came out with what I was expecting all along, my self-fulfilling prophecy: the breakup.

"For me," he began, "dating goes one of two ways. One way: I go out with a woman and I fall head over heels for her, I get very attached. It doesn't last long. The other way: I don't feel any chemistry whatsoever and I never see the woman again."

He paused.

"Yeah?" I prodded. I knew what was coming.

"With you," he said, "it's neither. I think we should just be friends."

He said he wanted me to know so that when we went out on my birthday I wouldn't try to kiss him.

Did he think I was unattractive? I couldn't help but wonder if knowing my past had turned him off.

"Is it because of my history?" I asked. I thought about Mitch. "Is it because I won't just hop into bed?"

"No," Jason said. "Not at all."

Again, I wasn't sure I believed him.

"I've never had such open and honest conversations as I've had with you," he continued. "Not with anyone, except maybe my best friend from high school, but definitely not with a woman."

"What's wrong with an open and honest conversation?" I asked.

"Nothing," Jason said. "That's my point. It's great."

"Why does that mean 'just friends'?" I asked.

In my mind, that kind of connection with a man was what led to physical intimacy. To me, physical and emotional intimacy weren't mutually exclusive. I wanted and expected both in a relationship. Even though I had some fears around sex I thought I could work through them with the right man.

"It just does," Jason said.

When we went ice-skating on my birthday, Jason insisted on paying my entrance and skate fees. Spending the afternoon together, Jason shared more personal information about his struggles. I reciprocally shared more of mine, but I was growing weary of his ways, confused by his intentions.

"It's interesting," Jason said, "how we're all kind of like damaged children who are searching within others for what our parents didn't give us. But the thing is, we'll never find what we lost."

"I'm not trying to find what I lost," I said. "That's impossible. And it's a recipe for disaster in a relationship."

I was trying to move on from my past, while I sensed Jason was at odds with the idea, as if he were treading water in the holes of his heart, which was what I'd done for many years.

After ice-skating, he drove me home and followed me inside my apartment to give me my birthday present, a dozen cans of Trader Joe's salmon. Over tea and cake in my kitchen, he told me that he was dating another woman. Actually, he clarified, he was dating two women, and he'd been dating them while he'd been dating me.

"I'm wondering if you might have any advice?" he said. "Since we're friends now?"

"I think it's time for you to leave," I said.

To Jason, emotional and physical chemistry were two separate concepts, two distinct experiences that never merged. In an email he sent a few days later, he said that this was "the peculiar thing" about him. He wrote: "In an ideal world they'd be together."

A part of me continued to mull over whether my history had been the ultimate clincher for Jason and if the rest of his explanation was just a load of bull. I considered whether the reason was that he saw me as "damaged goods." The reason was I wouldn't just jump in the sack. But I finally came to realize the reason wasn't my history. The reason was *me*: I was thirty-five years old, and, for the first time in my life, I was asking a man for a healthy romantic relationship.

I was seeking real, intimate love.

Womanhood

I ALWAYS THOUGHT I'd face major life crises, such as the loss of a job or a health scare or the decline and death of a parent, with the support of a boyfriend or husband. But as life would have it, I'd go through such rites of passage without a partner. In the process, what was missing from my life came into focus: I took a hard look at my priorities and goals surrounding love.

It was past time to reclaim my womanhood.

———————

At the time of my mother's ovarian cancer diagnosis, when she was sixty-five, she wanted to be a grandmother. I just wanted to be normal.

I was thirty-six years old and, as an adult, I'd never had a lover, a fact I was ashamed to admit and had divulged only to Dr. Ross. Unlike many sexual abuse survivors who become promiscuous in reaction to their experiences, I'd avoided sexual encounters. Sometimes, I wished to have been promiscuous; at least then, I believed, I'd be a sexually experienced woman, a mark of normalcy in the eyes of others. Although I wanted to be in a relationship and played out idealized romantic scenarios in my mind, the truth was that when it came to actually being with a man I felt like somebody's prey.

I equated sex with rape. When I was sexually abused, I was manipulated into acts that entailed the same genital body parts and motions as intercourse, but that was not the same thing, Dr. Ross said, as having sex. I was a de facto virgin.

But I didn't consider myself a virgin. I considered myself an anomaly.

I didn't know if my mother knew I wasn't having sex. All I knew was she wanted me to get married and have children. If I did, that would mean I was normal and that she was normal, like other women.

When I noticed a potential boyfriend looking at me with interest, I was convinced he'd pass me over once he saw through my superficial appearance: With my clothes on, I believed, I was false advertising. I imagined that once he saw me naked he'd view me as abnormal, in a light of lesser worth, because of what had happened to me when I was a child. What man, I thought, would want to be with a woman who'd had sexual experiences with her father? Only another abuser. And I didn't want a relationship with an abuser.

Six months before her cancer diagnosis, my mother told Russell that her life was "miserable" because she didn't have grandchildren as other women her age did.

Russell relayed the conversation to me: "I told her I wasn't going to be able to deliver," he said. He was a single gay man. My mother seemed to take this as a reason to excuse him. Cased closed, discussion over.

Continuing the lineage was my charge.

"You could meet someone in the next year or two," my mother encouraged me. She was positive. "You could have a baby by the time you're forty."

"Having children is important to me," I told her, though I didn't think she realized just how much, even though over the years, as my peers got married and gave birth, she'd frequently heard my discontent over my lack of a boyfriend and other voids in my life. I added, "The way you keep bringing up wanting grandchildren is painful for me."

"I don't mean for it to be *painful* for you," she said. "But I have a right to say what I want."

I swallowed my thoughts: *I wanted to grow up in a safe home, I had a right to that, but you didn't give me that. Yet I owe you grandchildren?* I didn't want to hurt her by saying something I'd regret, so I simply replied as gently and clinically as I could: "I'm working very hard in therapy to get my life together, but I don't know if I'm going to heal in time to find someone to marry and have children."

She proposed that I freeze my eggs. "It's just something to consider," she repeated, "so that you at least have an option."

Her sense of entitlement bothered me. I had enough trouble covering my rent, which my mother knew, so how did she think I could pay to freeze my eggs, and for whose benefit were my eggs?

I thought my mother blamed me for her lack of grandchildren, and I sometimes felt I deserved such blame. But in this moment, I wanted to shake her and
tell her that if she'd protected me when I was a girl, if she'd stopped the abuse,
perhaps I'd be "normal." I wouldn't have become riddled with problems surrounding intimacy, or now need to spend so much time and money on therapy
to fix myself. Perhaps I'd be in a relationship or married by this point in my life.
Perhaps she'd have her grandchildren.

These things were too difficult to say aloud. "I don't have the money to freeze
my eggs," I said instead. And my mother didn't offer monetary help.

I thought that in my mother's eyes I was a failure. "Normal" thirty-something
women bore children, if they hadn't already done so during their twenties.

———————

The truth was, despite my fears, I wanted to have sex. I desired to eventually
share my life with a partner and to create a life together with him. I wanted to
ultimately have a baby within a committed relationship, within a psychologically and financially stable home. I didn't want to replicate the family circumstances of my childhood. I wanted to make sure I was emotionally healthy
before raising a family, because I understood the consequences if I, as a mother,
was not.

I knew that not all women in stable, committed relationships chose to have
children. I also knew, from sitting in a reproductive specialist's waiting room
when I was in my late teens and early twenties, that many were not physically
capable. Beginning when I was fifteen, I suffered from irregular periods, a condition misdiagnosed first as adrenal hyperplasia (a congenital disorder) and then
as polycystic ovarian syndrome, only to finally, in my early thirties, have it get
chalked up to the traumatic stress of the sexual abuse I'd suffered as a girl. Years
before I uttered the truth, my body spoke of it. Once I began to face my past in
therapy, my cycles regulated.

At thirty-six, I was able-bodied. I despised my biological clock and the wom-
en's magazines that pointed out, with unrelenting persistence, that time was running out, if I was not already too late. Colleagues and acquaintances suggested

that if I ever wanted to have a child I should become a single mother, a "choice mom." I shouldn't wait, they said like an alarm, I had to do it *right now*.

But I was in no position to have a baby. I had a full-time teaching job, but I was on a yearly contract. I didn't have job security. I had no savings. I used any cash surplus I had from my monthly income to pay for my PTSD treatment. I attended individual and group therapy appointments multiple days a week, along with neurofeedback therapy, to cope with extensive anxiety and depression. I didn't have the kind of life necessary to provide for a baby. To me, there was no choice.

"I'm not going to have a child," I said, "just to have a child."

———

My mother wanted me to bear children, but she didn't want me to be a sexual woman.

When I told her that Mitch and I had broken up, she said, "Seeing him was a *mistake*," her tone striking the combination of admonishment and fear she used whenever we spoke not in theoretical terms but of my actual romantic life. This was about more than just the fact that Mitch wasn't Jewish.

"Men only want one thing," she reiterated.

———

In fifth grade, my teacher, Mrs. Trumani, had a contest to see how many "dollar words" our class could come up with. Each letter of a word was assigned a numerical amount corresponding to its placement in the alphabet. For example, the letter "A" equaled one cent, the letter "B" equaled two cents, and so forth. My contribution to the list was the word "Virgin." I remember how Mrs. Trumani came over to me, her hands like blinders, shielding the sides of her lips, as she mouthed just to me, "Virgin." She'd noticed that I'd posted it on the "dollar word" chart hanging on our classroom wall. I, along with my fellow ten- and eleven-year-old female classmates, had just seen the girls' guide to maturation film the previous week. Mrs. Trumani smiled as if it was our little secret, as if I was budding into a beautiful young woman. I felt my cheeks turn pink.

That afternoon I went home and asked my mother what a virgin was. She told me to look it up in our *Merriam-Webster* dictionary, which was located on the shelf in Russell's bedroom. Of course I already knew the definition, but I pretended I didn't. My mother sat on Russell's bed with the dictionary splayed across her lap as she told me, "It's a woman who's never been touched by a man." My body felt stiff and warm as she told me that a woman shouldn't allow herself to be touched by a man until she's married.

My mother never said the sexual abuse was my fault, but as I went through my PTSD recovery, I interpreted her reaction to my disclosure of the abuse as one that pointed to my culpability. I imagined she saw me as a willing and equal participant of a marital affair. I reflected on the time I was a teenager and my mother was hospitalized for a breast cancer scare: I was, as Dr. Tetley had said, in the role of "the little wife." I hadn't stopped my father from putting me in that position. I'd wounded my mother so deeply and as a consequence she developed cancer.

Part of me wondered if my badness was why my mother didn't stop the abuse all those years, not because she didn't know, but because she was angry with me, because my body had responded favorably to sexual touch, because part of me had liked it, because her husband had liked me.

Your father's face lights up when you walk into the room. He no longer "lit up" for her.

Part of me wondered if my mother developed a gynecological cancer because of our family's past, because I'd been sexually abused, because my father's ejaculate was somehow poisonous, because of all those years of denial, because I brought the truth out into the open by speaking and unleashing a lifetime of toxicity that then ran rampant inside my mother's body like a thousand assassins.

Months before my mother's diagnosis, during her yearly gynecological exam, a pelvic ultrasound showed "a white spot." Her doctor recommended she undergo an MRI to determine diagnosis. My mother, who'd always been proactive about her health, refused.

"I told them I couldn't," she explained to me five months later, long after she'd started developing the physical symptoms of ovarian cancer. "I'm claustrophobic," she rationalized. "I can't tolerate feeling like I'm in a coffin."

The late-stage carcinoma was thought to have begun in the fallopian tubes, the pathways from the ovaries to the uterus, where the egg and sperm meet for fertilization, where I came into being. If the egg doesn't become fertilized, it deteriorates and is removed from the body by the immune system, during the process of menstruation.

———

Just like my mother, I began menstruating when I was thirteen.

I was home from school during winter break, eating lunch with my mother and Russell, when my abdomen began to ache badly and I left the table to go to the bathroom. When I pulled down my pants I saw a deep brown-red blotch on my underwear. My heart raced.

"Mom!" I yelled. "Mom!"

She came rushing to the bathroom door.

"What is it?" she asked.

I let her in.

"I think I got my period," I said, showing her my underwear and then looking at the floor. Blood coming from that part of my body made my face turn hot. I saw it as a non-removable stain, an announcement to the world that I was a sexual being, that I was dirty.

My mother gasped with joy. "Oh, Tracy!"

"I know what happened!" Russell called from the kitchen table.

My mother washed my underwear, gave me a clean pair along with an Always pad, and pinched my cheeks.

"You've become a woman," she told me, her eyes enlivened. Then she called my father at his office to tell him the news.

That afternoon, for a long while I sat on my bed in my room with my knees drawn close, feeling a sense of danger. "You have to be very careful now to not get raped," I thought to myself, even as I blocked from my awareness the ongoing sexual abuse. "You could get pregnant." (Perhaps that was why my periods became so infrequent and my ovaries stopped releasing eggs all those months during all those years: My body was protecting me.)

That night, my father didn't come home until after I'd gone to bed, but when he did he came into my room with a box of Hershey's kisses and set them on my dresser. I could feel him staring at me as he stood there, his body blending in with the darkness. I thought he could see right through the blankets and my nightgown, to my sexual parts.

"How are you feeling?" he murmured.

"Okay," I whispered.

I could smell the chocolate, see the way the silver wrappers glistened like tears. My father tousled my hair with an uncomfortable brevity, gave me a quick peck on the top of my head, and then he pulled away, said "get some sleep," and left the room, and I lay back down in bed, feeling a little like a baby doll put back on the shelf or buried in the closet, beneath the new toys, too old to play such games now.

What was supposed to be a life symbol seemed to be a token of death.

———

A week after my mother's cancer diagnosis and the removal of her quarter- and dime-sized tumors, along with her ovaries, fallopian tubes, uterus, two lymph nodes, and part of her omentum, she revealed to me that her doctors had tested her for the BRCA1 and BRCA2 gene mutations, a genetic lineage common among Ashkenazi Jews.

She was positive for BRCA1.

We learned that from the day of her birth my mother's lifetime risk of developing cancer was high: Her chances of developing breast cancer were 87 percent versus the general public's 7 percent, and 44–66 percent for ovarian cancer versus the general public's 2 percent.

Because I might've inherited my mother's mutation, I decided to undergo my own BRCA genetic testing, as my gynecologist recommended I do for my own protection, for prevention: I didn't want to stick my head in the sand.

When I asked my mother for a copy of her BRCA genetic test results, which the cancer prevention clinic informed me I'd need to have in hand at my appointment, she hesitated.

"It's an invasion of my privacy," she stated over the phone.

I felt as if I were violating my mother with my request for information. At the same time, I felt betrayed by her desire to protect herself at my possible expense.

"But this is for my health," I said.

Since my mother hadn't signed the HIPAA release form, I knew that if she denied me her test results there'd be nothing I could do to get the information.

My mother always said that knowledge was power, and yet she frequently left me powerless. When she was rushed to the hospital for a bowel obstruction caused by scar tissue from her initial surgery, I was speaking with her on the phone from her gurney when she began vomiting uncontrollably and became unresponsive. I thought she was dying. I hung up and called the emergency room and insisted the doctor—*someone*—help her immediately. Later, my mother lashed out. She was angry because I had, in the process, spoken to her doctor. "*I* will tell you information," she raised her voice, "when *I* am ready to tell you!"

"But what if you're unable to tell me?" I asked, beginning to cry.

"Do you tell *me* everything?" she asked with a sharpness that made me shrink. I thought she was referring to the way I hadn't vocalized what was happening to me when I was a child, and to the way she felt that now, as an adult, I was withholding myself from her.

I thought she despised me.

"No," I answered, hearing my voice sound like a girl's.

"And why is *that*?" she countered.

Case closed. Discussion over.

For the first time, I saw a side of my mother I'd always known but had wanted to deny existed: Part of her was a bully. In hindsight, I understand her anger was most likely driven by her fear. Perhaps she was struggling not only with the possibility of losing her life but also with an unbearable remorse that she might have, unwittingly, passed along her fate to me. But at the time, on the receiving end of her harsh tones, I didn't feel her love. I only felt her hate.

I pressed my mother to send me a copy of her BRCA test results, reiterating that I needed them in order to have the genetic testing.

"What will you do if you have the mutation?" she demanded. "Will you have your breasts and ovaries removed?"

"I don't know," I said. I tried to separate myself from what felt like badgering. I really couldn't imagine what I'd do, not yet. All I knew was this was a matter of life and death, and I wanted to acquire whatever information I needed to protect myself, and my future. I was fighting to save my life.

"It's all a business, this testing," my mother practically spat over the phone. "They can find a pill to fix erectile dysfunction, but they can't find an adequate test to detect ovarian cancer?"

I listened to her express her rage. I thought it made her feel stronger, though I saw her becoming weaker. I wondered how she really felt about the loss of control over her body, the violation of the surgery, the profound grief she didn't share.

What I didn't share was my own worry that I'd inherited the BRCA mutation, and that I'd end up just like my mother. After all, ever since my teenaged years, people had frequently commented that my mother and I looked and sounded alike, which pleased my mother but didn't really please me. Aside from what I saw as my mother's physical attractiveness and her flair for writing and editing, as an adult I didn't want to resemble her, particularly her tragic life scope, her way of living—or, in this case, dying. When I was in high school, as we watched the mother-daughter pageant on television, my mother fantasized about the two of us as contestants. She turned to me and grinned: "Which one's the mother and which one's the daughter?"

"I don't want you to have to deal with this," my mother said before finally agreeing to send me a copy of her results, though I could still hear the resistance and resentment in her voice. I imagined she might be wondering, what if I'd been spared while she hadn't?

Would that be fair?

A few days later, my mother mailed me her pathology report instead of her genetic test results. When I called to let her know her mistake, she became flustered.

"I misunderstood what you wanted," she said.

When I mentioned the discrepancy to Dr. Ross during my next appointment, he suggested that perhaps this wasn't my mother's mistake at all but rather some deeper wish of hers to tell me the truth, to circumvent her own denial.

By now it was too close to my genetic testing appointment for my mother to mail me the information, so she read it to me over the phone.

"187DELAGBRCA1," she enunciated the numbers and letters as I wrote them on a piece of paper. Her voice was clear and sober. "Deleterious. Deadly."

Later, I examined my mother's pathology report. I read that her cancer was a "high grade peritoneal mullerian carcinoma, mixed transitional and clear cell type." In his cover letter, the pathologist described my mother as "the poor patient" with "clear cell carcinoma so beautifully seen on the slide." Although the letter was addressed to my mother's surgeon, and not to my mother, my mother had it in her possession. I knew she'd taken in his words because she'd underlined and circled in pen much of what he'd written. As I read the closing paragraph, I became angry, certain that such an objectification of my mother's body had only compounded her suffering: "Most interesting morphology and your slides are very well stained," the pathologist wrote. "I would be delighted if I could keep one . . . as it is such a good example of this form of carcinoma. I have taken the liberty of doing so on the hope that you do not mind getting superficial results."

To me, the pathologist was posturing as some kind of Dr. Frankenstein and I wanted to take down what I saw as his egomaniacal stance. I wrote a scathing letter in response, which I copied to my mother's surgeon and to the head of the pathology department, who'd been copied on the original report, recommending that in the future he watch his word choice, pointing out that there was a real person reading his letter from inside the body he so described.

Unexpectedly, I received a note of apology the following week from the pathologist, in which he explained that he'd been writing for a medical audience and that he understood from personal experience what it was like to have a family member stricken by cancer. The next time I saw my mother, I gave her the apology to keep. When she took the letter in her hands, I noticed the smallest tinge of a thankful smile spread across her lips and eyes.

Although my mother told me she was going to be fine, when my own gynecologist read the pathology report just before I went for my genetic appointment at a cancer prevention clinic located at a nearby hospital—I wanted to ask her medical opinion on my mother's (and in foresight of the testing, my own) prognosis—her countenance grew grave.

"I'm sorry to tell you," my gynecologist said, "that this is a very aggressive form of ovarian cancer that doesn't respond well to treatment. You should encourage your mother to do the things she wants to do in the time she has left."

I was shocked. I trusted my gynecologist. She'd been straight with me since my first appointment with her six years earlier, when I was thirty, when Dr. Ross referred me to her as a doctor who understood how to best approach and examine women who were coping with sexual trauma. I hadn't been able to have a pelvic exam; my body always closed down on the speculum as if it were a live wire. The pain was unbearable. I'd avoided doctors out of fear and shame. But this doctor was compassionate along with being knowledgeable. She supplied detailed anatomical information about my body, answered my medical questions with facts, and, after several appointments over the course of a year in which she slowly oriented my mind and body to the pelvic exam, she helped me move through my PTSD response in order to complete my first pap smear. She also answered my questions about sex.

My mother insisted that my gynecologist was wrong.

"My doctors aren't worried," she said testily. "And *they* are the specialists."

My mother was still working her job, going about her normal daily life (and, in fact, continued to do so until a few days before she died). At the time, I wondered if her doctors were really telling her she was going to be fine, or if she just didn't want to hear the truth. I didn't blame her.

I blamed myself. Whenever she was irascible, I heard in her voice a loathing for who I was, for what I'd been involved in as a child, for what I had done and not done as an adult, for the way that was all ending her life.

I thought that testing BRCA-positive would be my due recompense, and that consequently I'd never find a life partner, because I didn't deserve one.

———

A week later, I sat, feeling paralyzed, in the cancer prevention clinic. Caught in a whirlwind of past, present, and future losses, I focused on the sterile-white tile floor where my face and body reflected as an undefined mass, a gray blur. Turning for a moment to look over my shoulder, out the window, I peered at a park and tennis courts down below, devoid of people, flooded by rain. Staring out at the vast expanse of green, an uncommon sight in the city, I thought about what it would feel like for my body to smash through the glass and plummet to the ground.

As a prerequisite for my genetic test, a simple blood draw, I had to attend a one-hour meeting with a genetic counselor, a young brunette woman who delivered the facts as if she'd freshly memorized them for an exam: "187DelAg means deletion at gene 187," she said.

Seated across from me at a small conference room table, the counselor explained: Every gene has two copies. If you lose one to mutation, you have another copy so you're still ok, but if both are lost then cancer happens. You can lose a gene from environmental factors or by inheriting a mutation.

"There's a fifty percent chance you have inherited this mutation," she said. "It's the flip of a coin."

I knew that twenty-five percent—one-quarter—of girls become victims of sexual abuse, as I had. The chance that I'd inherited a gene mutation, a death-marker, was double.

The flip of a coin: yes or no. Life or death: If I tested positive for the mutation, my future, I concluded, would vanish.

Management included surveillance—ovarian ultrasound, the cancer-marker CA-125 test every six months, annual mammogram, yearly breast MRI, a clinical exam twice a year, prophylactic mastectomy, chemoprevention, and ovarian removal "after you have your children," the counselor stated, "between the ages of thirty-five and forty."

"But I'm already thirty-six," I said. Like a death announcement, it occurred to me that I might've missed my window.

I already thought the chances were slim that I might ever get married. As an adult, I'd never let a man see or touch my bare breasts. Now, I thought to myself, if I was marked by a genetic mutation, I might not ever be able to experience childbirth. I might not ever be what I thought it was to be "normal" as a woman.

At this point, I'd been in therapy for several years, working to wrap my mind around what had happened to me as a child, in my family, to understand how I'd isolated myself from relationships, narrowed my adult life. Every day, with every interaction, I struggled to overcome my inheritance, to reclaim myself, to live. But none of that could counter a gene mutation that would cause my premature death, which I could prevent only by 98 percent, according to the counselor, if I chose to have my sexual organs removed.

What I couldn't bear to face was the way I felt as if my intimate parts had already been taken.

My past flashed before me: I saw myself as a child, as my father and I spent our special time together in my bedroom or in our basement. I saw my mother sitting on the black-and-white pinstriped couch in our living room upstairs, reading the *New York Times*; I saw her as she lay across the hall, sleeping soundly in her and my father's bed, as if she were in a coma while I was being abused.

Denial blanketed our home.

"They call it the silent killer," the counselor said, her eyes leaving mine for the surface of her large diamond engagement ring, and then to the oval table, where she placed a large pink slip of paper on which my family tree was neatly printed. With her red pen, she circled names and traced the cancer line: my mother, her sister, my grandfather, his sister, their mother. Next to my name, she drew a question mark.

It was the flip of a coin, but it was more than that to me. I didn't want to live my mother's legacy. I didn't want to die as I thought she already had, in her soul, when I was being abused as a girl.

"By deciding to take this test you can forge a different path," the counselor said. "One of knowledge."

She led me, finally, to the phlebotomist. As my upper arm was tied with the tourniquet-like rubber band, I turned my head away so as not to see my vein bulge or the needle penetrate my skin. I held my breath, waiting to feel the prick, then counted through the brief sensation of stinging tightness until I heard the clink of the vial on the counter and the slap of the rubber releasing its hold.

Processing the result would take between one and three weeks. Then I'd have another appointment with the counselor, because, according to policy, such information was only to be disclosed in the presence of a professional.

I assumed the test would find me marked, doomed. My inner makeup could not be changed; the facts of my genes were out of my hands. I could do nothing but wait for the shoe to drop, anticipate the imminent end.

I left the clinic, the soles of my feet slap-slapping the wet pavement as I traveled the four blocks to the T, feeling like a girl running home to a mother who wasn't there. Forty-five minutes later, I reached my apartment, shut the door behind me and tried to catch my breath as my body went weak and I slumped down onto the living room floor, vomiting up sobs.

Hannah trotted over, meowing softly. She blotted my cheeks with her calico tail, then ran her nose across my forehead. We no longer lived in the house with Margaret and King Tut; Walter had died and Margaret and Dean and their youngest brother fought over what to do with the property. In the end, the house was sold to a couple who chose to demolish it so that they could build condos; they didn't even wait until I moved out before they began bulldozing. I lost the home I loved and moved into the only apartment I could find on short notice, a place my friends called "the garret," a tiny one-bedroom attic unit with miniature windows, slanted ceilings, a dwarf-sized refrigerator and matching sink. When the movers climbed the narrow, steep staircase that led from the old house's back belly, as if up a ladder, to the garret door, they commented that it must have once been the maid's quarters. Unable to fit my loveseat up the twisted stairs, I had to leave it behind, along with my writing desk and bookcases. As I examined my losses I wondered, what were my gains?

Letting my tears dampen Hannah's fur, I noticed how, once timid and withdrawn from her own life in an abusive home, she now flopped on her side to expose her pure white belly, to offer her sweet, healing affirmations. I wept for the salvaged life I saw for her, but thought was lost for me.

———

Anxiously awaiting my BRCA results, I visited my mother. She sat, looking frail and smaller than I'd remembered, on her condo deck, with an umbrella shading her full head of hair, which, she lamented, she would soon lose from undergoing chemotherapy.

She'd asked for me to bring along a story that I'd recently published in the *Southampton Review*, a nonfiction piece that chronicled our family drives out to the east end of Long Island for our summer vacations when I was a girl, portraying the way my father had tortured me in the car, and how my mother, sitting in the front passenger seat, asked my father to refrain from his behavior. He didn't. After a while, resigned, my mother turned her head to look out the side window—she was gone as my world went spinning.

The editor-in-chief of the *Southampton Review* had invited me to read my story at a publication launch in Southampton, Long Island, very close to the location of the scenes I'd written. I'd made arrangements to attend, but then a week prior to the launch my mother was first diagnosed with her cancer. I drove from Boston to the hospital in New York, where I found her post-surgery, sitting beside her gurney-like bed, eating her breakfast, her hospital gown like a large cloth napkin draped around her shoulders.

"Hi, Mom," I said, hearing my voice float outside my body, feeling a heavy pressure at the back of my mouth, as if my tongue were a quivering dam, holding back an overwhelming grief my mother hadn't invited.

"You're early," she said, as if she wasn't ready for me.

I approached to hug her and she stood, pushing herself up from the hospital chair. I wrapped my arms around her thinness, tucking my chin over her shoulder as I started to weep, unable to control myself, feeling my chest shake and thump against her collarbones, my muscles and bones crying *mommy, mommy*.

"It's okay, it's okay," she repeated softly through her own tearful gulps as she embraced me, then pulled herself back, standing stoically, as if none of it—the cancer, the surgery, the past, this interchange, our show of emotions—had ever happened.

Although I seriously considered canceling my trip to Southampton, distressed my mother would see my reading as an act of abandonment and betrayal (she encouraged me to publish my work at the same time she expressed discomfort, saying "nobody wants to read about that" whenever she heard that I was writing about my experiences in our family), I ultimately decided to go. My friends and Dr. Ross encouraged me: "You'll regret it for the rest of your life if you don't," they all said. And, in my heart, I knew they were right.

While battling flashbacks (on my way to the site of the reading I recognized some familiar landmarks from the site of the story) and a cold that had lodged itself in my throat, I read as clearly as I could to an auditorium full of strangers, feeling the heat of the light from above on my skin, hearing my voice launch from the silent interior of myself into a realm of others, my story like a highway connector, taking me out of my isolation and linking me to the world, from person to person.

When I finished, applause reverberated in the auditorium, through my gut, around my ribs and collarbones, before the affirming vibration spread down my arms and across my face. As the audience dispersed, a young man approached me at the podium and shook my hand.

"I was hooked by your story from start to finish," he said. I was taken aback by the way his eyes were so alive with interest. "You've inspired me to work on my own story," he continued. "Thank you for reading."

His reaction, contrary to my expectations, turned me speechless for several moments. For the first time, I believed I'd done something right by sharing my truth.

———

Now, just a couple of weeks later, I was sitting with my mother on her condo deck, worried she perceived I'd done something wrong. At her request for my story, I reluctantly handed it to her. She put on her glasses and pushed her chair back, the legs scraping against the dull gray slabs of condo deck wood beneath her feet. I watched as she fingered the edges of the journal pages. Her head bowed as her wide eyes moved back and forth across my words.

"You're going to read it *now?*" I asked, hoping she'd wait until after I was gone.

My mother's face turned toward me. "You don't want me to?" she asked with a touch of disbelief.

"It might be upsetting," I said, apprehensive about her reaction. "This might not be the time."

She held the pages tightly in her grasp, insisting, "I want to read it *now.*"

"Okay," I said, sitting back, letting go. This was my mother's decision, I reminded myself, this was my mother's choice, for which I was not responsible.

I stared at my fingertips, as if willing myself to disappear through the transparency of my nails, while my mother read in silence.

When she came to the end, she began to cry softly. Standing up, she linked her arms around my body, and, for a moment, hung on to me like a heavy, worn coat. My fingers rested lightly on her back.

Her voice came from a deep part of herself: "I'm so sorry," she said, "that I wasn't there for you."

Out of habit, I brushed her words aside. "It's okay," I said, trying to console her.

"No, it's not okay," she said, pulling back and sitting down, her blue eyes suddenly bright and looking directly into me. "You captured it accurately on the page," she spoke with clear certainty. She pointed her forefinger at me: "None of it was your fault."

I believed her.

Then she changed the subject, asking me how much it might cost to freeze my eggs, as if she'd said nothing, read nothing, at all. In the weeks and months that followed, she'd continue to exercise her trademark defensiveness and denial around the truth. But in that moment, I chose to linger at that window my mother had unlocked, to stop time, to sit with that fleeting peace, to open it within myself.

In that moment, I didn't know my future: My genetic test result was negative. I hadn't inherited my mother's legacy.

I was already free.

———————

In therapy, I began to face my unresolved fears around intimacy, sorting out the difference between what had happened to me as a girl and what I, as an adult, had a birthright to have: consensual sex.

I began to feel more comfortable about the idea of sharing the truth of my years of sexual isolation, and I told a couple of friends, as well as the members of a new therapy group I'd joined (in the later stages of PTSD recovery, I'd "graduated" from various trauma-based groups and was now in a coed relationship group for "regular" adult problems). A straight male member responded to my disclosure by saying, "I think it's understandable." Another said, "Why are you so hard on yourself? It's not your fault."

Initially, I thought maybe they were just being nice. I hadn't considered a positive reaction possible. Yet the truth is, everyone has issues they bring to relationships, but we are greater, more whole, than our struggles. We are all survivors of something. We can't change the past, but we have the power to decide whether our history will define our future.

The trajectory of my life had been irreparably changed by events that were beyond my control. But I had agency. I began to redefine "normal." I saw myself not as aberrant, but real. I was someone who had the tested ability to cope with life's challenges. I grieved the years and experiences I lost, the men I never got to know, the biological children I would likely never have. I no longer blamed myself for the wreckage; I learned to let go of the pain.

I started living, putting myself out there, not just in dating but in all facets of my life. There were times when I saw my past was at play and obstructing my view. But that was a normal, human struggle. I found the freedom to invite intimacy and love into my life, and to make a choice to have sex or not, based on my desire and self-respect.

I wasn't a wife or a mother, but for the first time in my life I felt like a woman.

Cats Aren't Kids

I WASN'T A stereotypical "spinster." I wasn't a "cat lady."

I was a volunteer at the Animal Rescue League, where my title was "feline friend": I fed and played with the shelter cats and cleaned their cages; I socialized the scared and angry ones so that they'd "show" better to the public for successful adoption.

One day, a seven-week-old kitten was delivered to the shelter by a Good Samaritan who saw this mere speck-like ball of orange and white fur thrown from a car driving under an overpass on I-93, a major highway in Boston.

The shelter staff named him Lil' Trooper, because he'd survived a terrible ordeal. According to the intake report, Lil' Trooper exhibited head trauma, possible brain damage, numerous abrasions, and a degloved lower lip. The left side of his neck, just under his ear, was half-eaten by fleas. His belly was full of worms.

When I heard about Lil' Trooper's traumatic time in the car, I recalled my own childhood experience with my father on the highway. Sadness seeped in my chest.

In the Old Testament, the Book of Samuel tells the story of Hannah, a grief-stricken barren woman, wife to Elkanah. Hannah, whose name in Hebrew translates in English to "beauty" and "passion," wants nothing more than to bear a child. She weeps to God for the ability to conceive a life. God sees Hannah's despair and grants her the ability to become pregnant. She gives birth to a son, whom she names Samuel, meaning "word of God."

For years after my PTSD diagnosis, I sat by myself in synagogue on Yom Kippur as the rabbi retold this story of faith in the face of impossibility, fullness in the realm of emptiness. The words on the page blurred as I mourned what I'd missed out on during my decades of emotional numbness and isolation, the kind of life I believed I might never have, due to my past. I thought about how I'd come to adopt Hannah when my life (and hers) was so barren. I contemplated her story, and mine, the voids and the struggle to hold on to faith.

————

At the start of my volunteer shift, I went to Lil' Trooper's cage and found him sitting in a cardboard litter box, covered in excrement and flea dirt, and surrounded by a pile of poop. A handwritten note taped to his cage door reported a lack of urination, warning of the possibility that the trauma might have caused a bladder rupture, which, if confirmed, would mean he'd be put down: euthanasia.

Like a ragged coat worn by the homeless, matted orange fur covered his back, draped over his shoulders, hooded his ears, skimmed his forehead in the fashion of an "M," colored the length of his nose, and dotted the upper tip of his chin. His limbs were as thin as my fingers. Pure whiteness spread across his chest like a bib, lightened his cheeks, and outlined his nose and yellow-brown eyes, which he fixed upon my face. I saw his pupils were dilated, consumed by terror. I observed his fear and his vulnerable body, and I saw a part of myself.

I saw the way I trembled as I opened the cage door and offered my hand.

Lil' Trooper sniffed cautiously. I touched his tiny forehead with my thumb, between his eyes, and rubbed very gently, the way Hannah liked me to do.

Lil' Trooper began to purr, sounding like a car motor. He stood up, climbed out of his litter box, and moved toward me. When he reached a clearing, closer to me, he rolled over on his back and dangled his paws in the air, showing me the proverbial cat sign: "Rub my belly, please."

He was affectionate to his core. Even with all that had happened to him, Lil' Trooper's soul had remained intact, unfaltering in his ardor for life. His desire to connect with another being, what seemed to be the salvation of his true self despite his trauma, enamored me with the transformative power of love. His ability to trust a person after the violent act one had committed against him unearthed my sense of faith.

I picked up Lil' Trooper, his tiny 1.8-pound body cupped between my palms, removed him from his cage, and lay him against my chest, where I felt the vibration of his deepest self mingling with my heart. In the face of my mother's cancer diagnosis, I was moved by the way this tiny little being reached for and embodied life.

"Hello, sweetness," I said. "What a sweetness."

Hannah was getting a little brother. After his medical clearance, I brought Lil' Trooper home. And I renamed him Sam.

Some people consider their pets their kids. I've never felt that way. But having them to mother and love has certainly been a life-changing gift.

CHAPTER 8

"I WANNA DANCE WITH SOMEBODY (WHO LOVES ME)"

Dear Future Life Partner,

Before I could share myself with you, I had to learn to love myself, and my body. In the process of reclaiming my womanhood, I realized I was navigating the world as a "disembodied" person—I'd cut off my awareness of my physicality; I walked around with my chest collapsed and my shoulders turned in, with my head tilted down and my hips tightly wound, until my muscles and joints were riddled with tension and pain. I stopped allowing myself to express my spirit through bodily movement for so long that I forgot I had the capability, or the desire.

On Sundays at the gym, I spied on the Zumba class from where I was exercising on the Stairmaster. I remembered how, when I was five, my mother would put a Disney album on the record player and I'd skip and hop and leap around our basement for hours, paying attention to nothing and no one but the music and the way I danced. I lived and breathed the rhythm of each moment, until the sexual abuse shut down my innocent play.

Weekly, for almost a year, I watched the Zumba class through the studio's glass walls, envying the women I saw, women of all different shapes, sizes, ages, and agilities, moving their bodies so passionately, so freely, to Latin rhythms. They danced combinations of cumbia, merengue, samba, and other routines choreographed and led by Alan, the instructor I overheard one of the trainers refer to as "the epitome of life force."

I regularly took cardio classes, from cycling to boot camp to kickboxing, so I knew I was physically fit enough for a high intensity hour. But I didn't know if I could take more than a few minutes of Zumba. I didn't know if I could allow myself to unlock my hips and shoulders and chest and heart, where I stored the violation and terror and humiliation of my girlhood. Still, I wanted to try the Zumba class.

One day, I mustered up the courage to go in.

I stood in the back of the room so as to not be noticed making what I anticipated would be a fool of myself. I'd left my contact lenses at home, on purpose, so that I wouldn't be able to see myself in the mirror, but I could still make out the shape of my body in the distance: my purple tank top, my black workout capris, my blonde hair up in a ponytail. I felt my legs and arms and insides begin to shake. I'd spent years in therapy psychologically processing the various angles and effects of my trauma, peeling away the layers, but my body still held my wounds.

I remembered how, in seventh grade, I was the uncool, uncoordinated girl trying out for the school dance team, unable to kick high or do splits, or move my body gracefully as the other girls did; I tried not to notice everyone watching as I attempted to do something I thought only the lucky and deserving could do: express oneself, belong somewhere. I tried my best but failed to move my tightly clenched body in the ways necessary to dance. I thought everyone could see that I wasn't normal and that that was why, after tryouts, I didn't make the cut.

"If it's your first time taking Zumba," Alan said, walking in front of the mirrors, facing us, "just keep moving and have fun. Don't worry about knowing what you're doing." Then he turned on a warm-up song: Ariana Grande's "Break Free."

I entertained the notion that my belief in my ability to Zumba (action verb) might be wrong, or at least changeable.

When the dancing began, I felt utterly uncoordinated and embarrassed. Worse, I felt panicked by the sudden rush of chills and tears as my body moved. But I didn't stop. I shut my eyes, felt the music, and listened to the lyrics: I'm stronger than I've been before! / This is the part when I break free / 'Cause I can't resist it no more!

Inside, I felt my five-year-old self starting to dance, freed. A new song began, and I felt my seventh grade self, and then other ages, getting up from the sidelines, where they'd sat for decades, joining in. Slowly, I reclaimed my essence, and my body. Over the course of a few months, I moved from the back of the room to the front, where I could see myself fully in the mirror.

A musical theater student, Alan was practically half my age yet his wise outlook and unconditional acceptance of everyone in the room made him seem years older.

He not only instructed us on the steps of each dance, but he also often shared his observations about life, including how we're frequently placed in positions of personal diminishment and how important it is to reclaim our space. Through his example, he gave us permission: "Take up space!" he ordered, flying across the room, cueing us to extend the reach of our arms. "Chest open and proud!"

The body was not an object to be debased, but a vehicle of our spirits to be celebrated, respected and honored.

"Do you feel sexy?" Alan shouted.

I did. I felt myself break free. I felt my joie de vivre. And I understood that no one could take that away from me.

I couldn't see it then, but a few years into the future I'd become a licensed Zumba instructor. I'd sign up to attend Zumba instructor auditions. When my nerves struck in front of judging eyes, I'd speak back to my old insecurities. I'd tell myself I had nothing to lose: I was simply putting myself out there; I was being me. To my surprise, I'd get hired to teach my own weekly class at a local gym—then two, then three.

I never thought it possible. But, as I'd find out, it, and so much more, was.

CHAPTER 9

YOU COMPLETE ME

Dear Future Life Partner,

I've sometimes asked myself if my life would be complete if we never met.

Living without a partner, I've mastered the art of aloneness. I've learned to do everything on my own. I'm quite self-sufficient and capable of handling life's challenges myself. Now I'm pursuing togetherness—the closeness, the sharing, the give-and-take support of long-term partnership. That's what I desire.

You know that line from the movie Jerry Maguire, *"You complete me"? I was in graduate school when the movie debuted, and, admittedly, I fell in love with the story. I still have the complimentary Academy of Motion Picture Arts and Sciences VHS tape that my screenwriting professor tossed my way during Oscar season. But that line? I dislike it, because it's not about partnership, it's about codependence. I don't see myself as incomplete without you, or you as incomplete without me. And I wouldn't want us to be. To me, being in partnership is different than needing a partner to "complete" you or your life: You are, I am, already whole. If we go into a relationship thinking otherwise, if we're looking to each other to fill a hole, we're setting ourselves up for failure.*

I know, how can I really understand what healthy partnership is if I haven't ever had a long-term partner? I've wondered why my coupled friends, of both genders, say that I give good relationship advice. Recently, I told my friend James, who was having relationship difficulties, to just take my thoughts with a grain of salt, because, given my lack of a relationship history, I'm obviously no expert. James called me on my self-critical remark and debunked it by pointing out how much experience I've had with many different kinds of relationships. I've also gleaned a lot through watching my friends date, marry, and divorce.

Many people can't bear to be alone—they latch onto any warm body, no matter the price. They stay in loveless, unfulfilling "partnerships" for years because they feel they need the other person in some way. After a breakup, they don't know what to do with themselves, how to get through the day or the week without another person to fill the space. They can't even fathom a few months without a significant other, let alone longer. They can't imagine how I've survived decades of singledom. But I have, and maybe I'm better prepared for something lasting because of it.

When we're going through hell, it's hard to see a silver lining. And yet for me, there have been real silver linings amidst the challenges and pain in my life. As I'll describe next, dealing with the loss of my mother without a partner, I learned how a higher kind of love allows us to transcend our relationship stumbling blocks and helps us to feel less alone in the process. I also learned how important it is to not idealize potential partners and relationships. Dating is hard work and the other person may not be up to the task, which isn't a reflection of your worthiness. Sometimes finding the love of your life is simply a fact of mutual rapport, timing, and luck.

What I'm about to share with you has to do with my process of moving on, closing the chapter on my younger life, letting those years go to their "resting place," which became the unexpected key to opening a new door and stepping into a new way of being, one of my own empowered creation.

But first I hit rock bottom.

Greatest Love of All

ALTHOUGH I'D ALWAYS assumed that when it came time to cope with the death of a parent I'd have a husband by my side for support, that wasn't where my life was at when my mother was declining. And, during that period, showing my best self to a potential boyfriend was difficult. I worried about appearing preoccupied, about being unable to concentrate on our conversation. I didn't want to burden a stranger or scare him away with my "mother lode." A budding relationship wasn't the time or place to share such heaviness, and, in the face of impending loss, lightness didn't come easy. I was convinced a potential boyfriend wouldn't want to get involved with someone in my situation—too messy. Truth be told, I wasn't sure, if the tables were turned, if I'd be gung-ho about the prospect myself. A dying parent can add a lot of interpersonal strain to a relationship that isn't yet on its feet.

I didn't want to embark on a new relationship only to see it dissolve. Already, someone I'd considered a good friend had withdrawn because my state of mind during my mother's illness was too taxing for her (ultimately, our friendship ended). They say a crisis reveals a person's true colors. My friend depended on me to be a rock, and she couldn't cope with my vulnerability, anxiety, and grief. She had a conflict-ridden relationship with her own (living) mother, one that caused her chronic depression, and my circumstances likely hit close to home. Though I was reasonably hurt when she wouldn't even acknowledge me when we passed each other on the street, I didn't blame her. I blamed myself for my choice of friends.

In the process of losing my mother, I realized who my true friends were. I had, in the years since my PTSD diagnosis, shed a lot of people from my life who really were nothing more than users. Now, at thirty-seven, as I let go of my few remaining unhealthy connections, I was developing more genuine friendships, but they were so new I was afraid such people would disappear if I leaned on them with an issue many hadn't yet coped with themselves. Trusting them took time, and so, aside from therapy, I mostly dealt with my mother's illness in the way I'd dealt with the other hard times in my life: alone.

Just as I needed to sever ties with my father in order to move forward in my love life, I had to break away from my toxic relationship with my mother and her damaging beliefs. Paradoxically, her illness loosened the boundary I'd enforced between us since my PTSD diagnosis, which gave me the chance to come to terms with my complicated love for her.

———

When she first began chemotherapy, my mother bought a wig and had her hairdresser color it close to her natural shade and cut it so that it matched her usual length. The wig's style was thin and straight, the opposite of my mother's curly crop, but she was pleased with it. The first time she wore the wig to the office, her coworkers gathered around and showered her with compliments.

"They said they liked my new style," my mother told me over the phone. "But I got a little nervous when someone tried to touch it."

They didn't know she had cancer, and she wanted to keep it that way.

When I visited, she wore a decorative scarf instead of the wig. A month after her first series of chemotherapy treatments ended, she led me to her bathroom mirror where she removed her scarf and showed me how soft patches of peach fuzz were starting to appear on her scalp, a sign that her hair was returning.

I felt queasy at the sight of her bare head. I wanted to look the other way, but I didn't, because I knew she needed me to see. At the same time, I understood that she wanted me to not see the truth that was reflecting back at us.

"That's great, Mom," I said as I watched her admiring herself in the mirror with a kind of morbid fascination that disturbed me. I thought she looked like a prisoner in a concentration camp.

Three months later my mother's hair had regrown, but she continued to wear the wig to work in order to keep people from knowing about the truth, even though she complained to me about how constricting the wig had become with a full head of her own curls underneath.

Soon after, my mother felt a lump between her legs. She went to the doctor, who ordered a PET scan.

"It lit up to a five," my mother reported over the phone, referring to the SUV "standardized uptake value," the numerical level of metabolic activity designated by the PET scan. The SUV typically ranges from zero to fifteen, with anything above 2.5 indicating metastases in the scanned area. "I don't know what it is."

"Maybe it's just a cyst," I said, bending my voice into as hopeful a tone as I could. I recognized my attempt to participate in my mother's denial, but I thought, given our ongoing tensions, it was better to try to appease and soothe her, particularly because she was sick. I didn't want to cause her further stress. I wanted her to get well. I also didn't want the bully part of her to emerge as it did whenever I tried to discuss reality.

"No," my mother insisted. "It's hard. A cyst wouldn't be hard. And I've felt strange for a bit."

"What do you mean 'strange'?" I asked.

"I don't know," she said, becoming irritated. "The surgeon will remove the lymph nodes and do a biopsy and then we'll find out what it is. He said at that point I could have more chemo."

"So he's saying it's a tumor?" I asked.

My mother exhaled sharply into the phone. "I don't like you accusing me of withholding information when I'm not," she said. "I'm telling you the *truth*."

"I was just asking a question," I said. "I'm your daughter. I love you. I'm concerned."

"I have to do this *my* way," she said. "I deal with things piecemeal. You always have to know everything. How dare you tell me that I withhold information from you!"

I hadn't wanted to go to this place with my mother—I'd wanted to honor her privacy without compromising the line between truth and denial—but I got caught up in my need for the facts, for transparency.

"For months," I said, "you withheld the fact that your gynecologist saw a spot on your ultrasound and that you had physical symptoms. I didn't know anything until you told me four days beforehand that you were having major surgery." I was tired of being blamed. I wanted my mother to hold herself accountable. I continued, "And then you refused to put me on the contact list for the doctor."

She'd put Russell's name on the list, but under duress he couldn't hold the information the gynecologic oncologist surgeon relayed to him during and immediately after the surgery; Russell became confused about the facts and passed along to me some incorrect information—he understood that our mother had cancer but he couldn't retain the specifics, such as the extent and location of tumors, the specific diagnosis and prognosis.

"I only put your brother on the list because he was there," she said. "If you were there, you'd have been on the list."

It was my fault. It was always my fault. I wasn't there. I was in the middle of teaching a two-week summer seminar over four hours away from the hospital. I'd asked my mother if she wanted me to be with her for the surgery and she said no. I wasn't sure if she was being honest, but I decided it best to respect her wish; I knew that probing her further about whether or not she was telling me the truth would only provoke her. Also, I didn't know how I'd get a substitute teacher for my seminar—my summer boss wasn't flexible and if I didn't show to class I'd lose the gig, along with the funds I needed to pay my next month's rent. Russell was more financially secure and able to take family leave from his job without penalty. Several times during and after the surgery, I was on the phone with him for updates. Then, that weekend, when Russell returned to work, I drove from Boston to the hospital in New York to take my mother home.

My mother's surgery for the newfound lump was scheduled for early April, in the middle of my spring teaching semester, when my employment situation had turned quite tenuous. Despite many years of excellent reviews, in the midst of politically driven tensions, I'd been asked to reapply for my position, and so I didn't want to cancel class unless it was absolutely necessary; I didn't want to give my boss a reason to terminate me. Absences, whatever the cause, were severely frowned upon.

My mother said that neither Russell nor I needed to be there; one of her college friends would be driving her to the hospital, and her local widowed friend Phyllis would be picking her up the following day to take her home.

Russell offered to be there anyway, but my mother emphatically told him no, though she changed her mind a day before the surgery. Unable to arrange to go that very instant, Russell arrived just before she went into the operating room.

The truth is, I felt guilty at the same time I felt relieved that I wasn't there.

During her recovery, my mother hesitated to share the updated details of her condition. I thought maybe it was just too painful for her to speak of it aloud. In a genuine attempt to alleviate her stress around disclosing difficult information, I offered to speak directly with her doctor. She took my gesture as an attempt to undermine rather than help her. I'd overstepped my bounds. "You've made me feel incompetent," she snapped.

A week later, when the test results were in and positive for cancer, my mother focused on how I'd wronged her. "The other day on the phone you forced me to tell you things I didn't want to."

"What things?" I asked.

"About the support group," she said.

She'd mentioned she was considering joining a support group for women with ovarian cancer. My response had been perfunctory: I said I thought it was a good idea and I asked what organization or person ran it. Ultimately, she decided she didn't want to go.

"If you didn't want to tell me about the group," I said, raising my voice, "then you shouldn't have told me."

"Then what would we talk about?" she exclaimed.

I felt caught in a battle of words, verbally dueling with my mother to determine who was to blame.

"We wouldn't," I said. "We'd end the phone call. Maybe that's what we should do from now on."

"You make up all these rules," she said. "And I can't keep them straight!"

I felt as if my mother was flailing in quicksand—she seemed to want me to save her at the same time I thought she wanted to pull me in. She was sinking, and I was to go down with her. I knew I had to disengage, but I didn't want to leave my mother helpless.

In truth, I was grieving the loss of my mother before her physical death. I'd been grieving her absence for decades. In my thirties, I felt she'd exiled me from her life—or had I been the one to leave her? The more I healed from the past, the more I stepped out of her world and into a healthier one, leaving behind the beliefs I'd inherited from her about how to navigate daily life, core beliefs that had foiled my attempts to cultivate relationships—with boyfriends, with friends, with employers, and, at the core, with myself—the more my mother dug in her heels, refusing to meet me where I was, and the further away she seemed. I wished to be closer to her, but if I wanted to have her, I couldn't have me. I wondered if my mother was dying because I was starting to authentically live.

The situation felt irremediable. I told her I needed to get off the phone.

"Alright," she said. "I'll speak with you in a few days."

We finished our call with the phrase we always used to end our conversations, no matter the mood:

"I love you," my mother said, though she sounded aggrieved.

"I love you, too," I said, feeling desperate for her to believe me, for us to finally connect.

I studied the soft undersides of my wrists, tracing the squiggly bruise-blue veins with my eyes. I thought maybe I'd been unfair or behaved with a lack of lovingness toward my mother. That was, after all, how she seemed to view our encounters. Perhaps I was a horrible daughter, as Donna had said I was when my father was sick.

I thought about how easy it might be to cut myself, or step in front of an oncoming car or train, to end my pain—and my mother's.

I wondered if my mother wanted to die. For a time, I did.

———————

This was one of the lowest periods of my life.

My boss notified me that my department was no longer pursuing my candidacy for my position. They were pursuing someone else who would take my job starting in the next academic year, my boss said, someone he labeled "more qualified." I'd accrued nine years of full-time teaching and administrative experience. My replacement was a graduate student who'd taught part-time in our department for one semester, a younger woman I'd trained.

With the prospect of unemployment, I didn't know how I was going to cover my rent and basic bills for the short- or long-term. Now I'd also have to pay for my health insurance premiums. I saw my life as one of complete failure. I saw my peers living stable and established lives: Sure, they had their problems, but most had secure employment, owned homes, were married, and were raising children, which were to me age-expected milestones I hadn't reached and thought I possibly never would. I remembered how, in my graduate screenwriting class, our professor often reminded us that a character who doesn't move forward has no purpose in the story; such a character is therefore generally killed off or eliminated altogether. I thought I was such a person. What I didn't see was that one's life status wasn't the only way of measuring progress.

"I'm not going to let you end up on the street," my mother said when I told her about my impending job loss. But she didn't offer to lend me money, and I didn't ask. I'd only once asked her for a loan, when I moved back to Boston and I didn't have enough money to pay for a required security deposit in addition to first and last month's rent for my studio apartment. At that time, she declined: "Lending money changes relationships," she said. "You'll have to ask your father."

I began to have trouble getting out of bed in the morning. I was the person everyone always said could "handle anything." I'd grown exhausted from the pressure. I was the one friends and family counted on to be the rock, to bounce back, to "be okay" no matter what. But I wasn't okay. I questioned whether any of the professional and psychological work I'd done over the past several years to improve myself and my life circumstances held any value. I saw everything I'd worked to build falling apart, unraveling, becoming null and void. I wondered if my life might get cut short by a fatal disease in the way it was happening to my mother, or if I'd die due to an accident or crime, before I ever really lived. Some days I thought that's what I deserved.

I told Dr. Ross I was feeling suicidal.

"I've worked really hard in therapy for years now, and my life hasn't changed," I said.

"That's not true," Dr. Ross said. "A lot has changed."

"Not enough," I said. "No matter how hard I try, I can't seem to catch up to everyone else."

"No, you can't catch up," Dr. Ross said. "You experienced something terrible, and the effects are real. Your life is never going to be what it would've been."

As much as I didn't want to, I had to accept this truth. All I could do was put one foot in front of the other and see what life might have in store. The problem was, I assumed there was nothing but more loss and disappointment ahead.

"I'm so tired of trying and failing to make things work," I said.

"Why don't you let your life unfold?" Dr. Ross asked.

"Because," I said, brushing away tears, "I'm afraid I'll find out that I don't have one."

Dr. Ross leaned forward. "Therapy can't get you a good job or a boyfriend or a healthy set of parents," he said. "There are a lot of variables in life, and no guarantees, but I *can* guarantee that if you didn't do this work your chances of living a fulfilling life would be quite low. You'd be nonfunctioning. But you're not. You're not like those women in that first trauma skills group you were in who were coloring."

I knew he was right, but I felt so weary.

Dr. Ross looked me square in the face. "Do I need to worry about you harming yourself?" he asked.

I noticed his olive eyes, the kindness and care in them.

"No," I said. I wouldn't actually do something to hurt myself. If I felt I was on the verge, I'd check myself into the emergency room.

"Are you sure?" he asked.

"Yes," I said.

"I'd be very upset if I heard that you killed yourself," he said gently. "I don't think you realize how upset I would feel."

I could tell by the sound of his voice and the way he tilted his head that when he said "upset" he didn't mean "angry." He meant "sad."

For the first time since I'd begun to face my past, I felt I mattered to someone—not for what I could do for them, but simply because I was me.

———

In order to prevent a major worsening of my depression, I carefully maneuvered the logistics of my visits with my mother, who lived three-and-a-half hours away, though I still had setbacks with each trip. I had, for a ten-month period of time before my mother's illness, refrained from visiting her (I still spoke with her by phone weekly), a period of time Dr. Ross called "a moratorium," to stabilize my mental health, even though my decision caused my mother to become even more upset with me. Visits with her sent me into depressive episodes. Now, I devised a travel plan for self-care: I drove to my mother's condo early in the morning, stayed for a few hours, and returned to my apartment before dark. I bargained with myself: I could deal with the stress of spending time with my mother if I could be in my own space at the end of the day. I told my mother I was unable to stay overnight because of my PTSD—in her condo, there were too many reminders of my childhood, including my father's fortieth birthday video gift that she still kept on top of the television set (I asked that she remove it before my next visit; she agreed, without protest—"I didn't even realize it was there," she said, as if my request had caused her to come out of the fog of a dream). I told my mother I needed to be in my own surroundings at night. She told me she understood, but when it was time for me to leave, she sighed and said gruffly, "Four hours doesn't do it for me."

It was as if I'd slapped her in the face. Anything I did to take care of myself or heal or grow was an offense. Once, a few years earlier, when I told her I thought I might want to spend Thanksgiving with a new friend, she forbade me: "You can spend time with other people after I'm gone," she said, referring to her future death (she was physically healthy at the time). "What if I want to spend a holiday with my husband's family?" I asked. "What husband?" she retorted. Her harsh words for me were plentiful, and yet I always minimized them, not wanting to believe this bullying voice was really my mother. For a long time, it was easier to take in her critical statements, let them press on me like sore bruise after bruise, and believe I'd done something to warrant them, than to draw a line, to say, "Stop, you're hurting me."

"I'm doing all that I can," I told her now, "but I have PTSD and I have to take care of myself. It would've been nice if you said you appreciated my visit. Four hours is all I can do."

"Is there anything else?" she asked brusquely.

"No," I said.

I didn't think she'd heard me. I suspected she'd heard my father instead: In her ears, I was her abuser, beating her down. Expressing my thoughts and feelings only worsened her pain.

———————

Two months later, my mother's barbed tone turned toward defeat.

"I no longer have joy in my life," she said over the phone.

Her statement was so simple and truthful and human that, rather than eliciting my anger, I was surprised to feel a sense of compassion toward her. I don't quite understand how it happened—perhaps it was a cumulative effect of my healing—but I found myself accepting my mother, her limitations, and letting go of my insistence that she be different. I stopped fighting the reality of who she was. I saw beyond her biting missives. That doesn't mean I excused her behavior; rather, it was about letting go of my own suffering in the midst of my mother's shortcomings.

My mother was suffering. She'd left her editorial post at the book publisher for a full-time position in publications at a university when I was twenty-six. She lost that job after she'd dedicated herself there just short of ten years, which was also just short of a retirement package eligibility threshold, when her position was phased out. Just before her cancer diagnosis, she began collecting partial unemployment while tutoring writing part-time at a community college near her condo. Her inquiries and interviews for full-time jobs never led to hiring. Now, her unemployment insurance was running out. On top of that, she said she could no longer take the long walks she'd always enjoyed at her condo complex, because she'd started to become short of breath, particularly when climbing the small paved hill that led the way out of her unit's cluster cul-de-sac. She complained of pain and swelling around her neck and left collarbone.

"What do you think is causing that?" I asked.

"I don't know," she said, sounding resigned rather than defensive. "I'll have another scan soon and then I'll find out."

I wanted to lift her spirits. "Do you ever think about getting back to writing?" I asked. "You used to love doing that." In her mid-thirties, my mother enrolled in a master's program in creative writing. She won a prestigious award for her poetry and published two essays in the *New York Times* about her strained relationship with her ailing mother, my grandmother. She stopped writing in her forties, a couple of years after my grandmother's death, when the tension between her and my father escalated and her reliance upon silence seemed to seal up her heart along with her creativity.

"Sometimes," she replied. "But right now I don't have the energy. Maybe I'll enroll in a memoir workshop in the fall."

"I bet you'd really like that," I said.

"Yeah," she sighed. "Well, I don't know."

I wanted my mother to retrieve what was once her love, to hold on to it like a buoy. I thought she could transcend what was killing her. I thought she could heal, as I was doing. Perhaps I was deluding myself, holding out a kind of hope that my mother and I could heal together and, in the process, reconcile.

"I've started to pray," she told me. "I know that may sound strange."

"It doesn't sound strange," I said.

"I've started to talk to God," she elaborated. "And Aunt Miriam. I ask them for a sign to let me know I'm not alone." Aunt Miriam was my late great-aunt, someone my mother had been closer to than her own mother.

"Do they answer?" I asked. I thought maybe I could do something for my mother: I could affirm and honor her from the place where she was. I could be her companion along her journey toward death. I knew my mother had always felt profound aloneness in her life. In my twenties, when my mother's remaining living sister died she cried, "They all hate me! They all left me!" She was referring to the family of her childhood: her parents and siblings, now physically all gone, though they'd been figuratively lost to her years before. My mother never came to terms with her losses; instead, she let each eat away at her, until there was hardly any of her left. This was her great well of pain, which she'd passed on to me since way before I was old enough to know it.

"In late winter I asked God to send me a sign," she said. "And when I looked out the kitchen window there was a flower in full bloom. And then I asked Aunt Miriam to send me a sign, and when I got into the car there was a foreign coin on the seat." She paused and laughed nervously for a moment. "Do you think I'm crazy?"

"No," I said. I noticed my heart was opening. Deep inside, I felt my compassion flowering into a kind of love beyond myself, a forgiveness I never thought I'd feel. "I don't think you're crazy at all."

———————

A few days later, my mother called to tell me that tests showed the cancer had made its way into the lymph nodes of her left armpit and neck. She had a blood clot, possibly more than one, between her clavicle and shoulder. That was why she had the swelling and pain.

I was puzzled as to why the doctor didn't keep her in the hospital after finding the blood clot, but I wondered if that was my mother's decision. She went home with Coumadin. She said that her periodic shortness of breath was "probably due to anxiety." But I had a bad feeling. Although I'd planned to visit her in the coming weeks, something in my gut told me not to wait. I wanted to talk with her in person about this newfound feeling of forgiveness that I felt growing within me.

———————

"What do most adult children do when their parent is very sick? They visit that parent, they help out," Dr. Ross said when I told him I was going to visit my mother. "But with your mother, it's complicated. I'm just concerned that you'll go into an emotional tailspin afterward. We know from experience that spending time with her tends to do that."

"I know," I said. "I'm worried about that, too. But I don't think she's going to be alive for very much longer, and I don't want to have any regrets."

Dr. Ross understood. "Tell me about this feeling of forgiveness," he said. "What's it like for you?"

I never thought I'd say so, but it felt freeing. I thought if I could tell my mother I forgave her, I could not only free myself, but free her, too.

She told me not to come.

"There's no *urgency*," she stressed over the phone. "I have a lot to do—laundry, cleaning, food shopping."

"I can help you with that," I said.

"I can do it myself," she answered.

My mother's self-sufficiency wasn't a healthy independence—she pushed people away. "I'll just keep you company then," I offered.

"We're having a *hurricane*," she insisted.

"Not until Sunday," I cited the official Hurricane Irene forecast. "I'll come Friday."

"But I want to *enjoy* your visit," my mother said petulantly. "You're only going to stay for four hours. It's going to be *rushed*."

"I plan to stay overnight," I said.

"But you said you can't do that," my mother said.

"It's no big deal." I heard my voice outside myself. Frankly, I wasn't sure how I was going to mentally get through such a visit, but I felt guided by something much bigger and deeper than my PTSD, something in my soul that was urging me to *go, go*.

"Look," I said, "the only reason I won't come is if you really want to be alone this weekend. I'll respect your wish if that is the case, but otherwise I'd like to spend time with you."

As if I'd flipped a switch, my mother's tone changed to one of childlike contentment. "Okay," she said. "I'd like it if you were to come."

Yellow jackets swarmed around us on the deck where my mother sipped a glass of iced seltzer with a slice of lemon. I pulled up a chair beside her at the gridiron table. I thought about the time I was there one year earlier, sitting across from her after her initial surgery and cancer diagnosis, handing her the story I'd published, the one she'd requested. I thought about how she'd read it and told me I'd written about the experience accurately, how she said she was sorry. In the weeks and months that followed, however, she reverted back to denial, and disavowal. I was writing a book about adopting Hannah and recovering from PTSD, and, because I'd never filed a police report and my father had never been arrested for or convicted of the crimes I alleged he'd committed, my literary agent recommended that I ask my mother to write a letter stating the abuse had occurred, for my own legal protection. My mother refused: "I believe that it happened," she said. "But I never saw it with my eyes, so I can't say that it occurred."

It took time for my forgiveness to unfurl, to embody a definition that I employed. I didn't subscribe to the kind of forgiveness that absolves someone of criminal wrongdoing or that is dispensed in the name of a higher power. I didn't believe in the validity of "forgive and forget." I didn't forgive my mother because she asked that I forgive, and she had asked me several times after I first told her about the abuse. My forgiveness wasn't about exoneration. My forgiveness was about letting go of my resentment toward my mother and my unmet wish for her to be different, to make the past and its effects on my life different.

On the deck, my mother spoke anxiously about her spreading cancer, her thoughts taking flight like the tiny bees that appeared in front of our faces. She swatted away the stinging intrusions with the backs of her hands.

"When's the surgery going to be?" I asked.

My mother shushed me, her eyes widening with concern. "Lower your voice," she whispered, afraid the neighbors would hear. She waved a yellow jacket away from her line of vision. "There isn't going to be any surgery," she continued. "You can't mess around with that area, the jugular is there."

Although I didn't say so, I wondered if the location was truly inoperable or if this was her way of telling me she'd made a decision to stop treatment, to let go.

"I'm not giving up," she said.

Was she telling me the truth? She listed her options: She could try another kind of chemotherapy, the third "cocktail" since her diagnosis; or, she could have radiation, which could shrink the tumors. There were too many "coulds" and my mother wanted a definite.

Her voice went up and down like a yo-yo: "They can't guarantee that any of it will work," she said, throwing up her hands. "I'm lucky," she glanced at me, "that the cancer is only in the lymph nodes, not in any major organs." But, as I'd find out after her death, when I'd discover a thick file of test results she'd kept in her possession, that wasn't true: The cancer was all over her body, including the center of her heart. She looked down at her lap, pursed her lips and sighed. She said soberly, softly, as if to herself, "I never thought this would happen."

Then she didn't want to discuss it any further: case closed, discussion over.

I took out my laptop and loaded some videos of Hannah and Sam playing in the garret. My mother's countenance lightened. She smiled and laughed lightly. She pointed to Hannah, clucking her tongue with a motherly affection I rarely heard: "She's still so cautious!"

That evening, my mother sat in our old recliner chair from the house where I grew up. Her hands were clasped in her lap, and her eyes were becoming heavy. Positioned across the room on one of my late grandmother's old red sofa chairs, I felt as if I were poised on the edge of the deep end of a pool, afraid but ready to dive in.

"Remember last summer," I began, "when you read my story, how you said you were sorry that you weren't there for me?"

The lamplight glowed like a halo around my mother's head as she turned and looked in my direction.

"Yes," she said.

"I appreciated that you apologized," I said. "It's taken me a long time, but I've come to forgive you."

My mother nodded. "I'm glad to hear it," she said quickly, unfeelingly, before her tone pushed back, "because I want you to *move on*."

No, no—my voice got caught in my throat. I took a breath.

"It's not about moving on," I said. "It's about forgiveness."

Forgiveness: I wanted her to take this in. *This is real*, I wanted to insist. I wanted my words to reach her soundproofed heart. I wanted to feel some kind of release, resolution.

"I forgive you," I said again, trying to penetrate a thick numbness I felt had enveloped the room.

And then I realized I'd set myself up for failure: For my mother to take in and accept my forgiveness, she'd have to take in and accept that she'd done anything wrong. She'd have to stop her flip-flopping. She'd have to look the cold hard truth in the face.

"If I had known," she said, "I would have done something."

Then she changed the subject, as if I hadn't said a word, as if none of it had ever happened.

———————

That night, after my mother went to bed, I sat surrounded by the physical reminders of my childhood: the 1980s television set from our old basement, with the broken VCR atop; the chair where my father once sat with me perched on his lap; the old record player, which hadn't been capable of spinning a forty-five for over twenty years—when I was a girl, every Saturday my mother polished the wood finish until it captured our faces in dull reflection.

I was immersed in the world of my past, that place where my body and mind had once resided, where down was up, where everything wrong seemed perfectly right because no one, especially my mother, batted an eye. I'd worked for years in therapy to get myself out of that realm, to orient myself to the truth, to enter a world beyond my victimhood. Now I was in what felt like an open grave.

My mother had dressed the air mattress I was to sleep on with the sheets of my teenage years. I didn't object. I lied down and shut my eyes. I focused on a safe place in my mind, as I'd practiced in therapy, to ground myself. But as I tossed and turned under the same covers in which I was once abused, triggers overwhelmed me.

I must have dozed off because suddenly I awoke to find myself sweating, my limbs thrashing, my heart pounding. I couldn't catch my breath. Only part of my mind was registering reality: *You're having a panic attack.* As I'd done all those nights of my childhood, I used my thoughts to soothe, to smooth over the truth, to wrap myself in a blanket of safety: *This isn't real, this is just a bad dream.* A nightmare.

After what seemed to be an eternity, the sun finally rose, ending the dark terror of night.

It was Saturday morning, and while I waited for my mother to emerge from her bedroom, where the door was shut down the hall, I quit the mattress and walked around the living room as if it were a museum, slowly making my way to a corner bureau on which my mother kept two framed photos of my brother and me as small children—in one I was a girl of three; in the other, I was nine. In the past, when I saw these pictures, I saw only pain in the faces of those girls but this morning they appeared to be smiling as if they'd been freed: her, and her. Me.

Perhaps, I thought, forgiving my mother had set something positive in motion, regardless of her reaction.

———————

My mother finally emerged from her bedroom, wearing her bathrobe and Isotoner slippers, moving unusually slow as she made her way into the kitchen to prepare breakfast: For years, she'd practiced a methodical daily rotation: Saturday breakfast was oatmeal with fruit and an English muffin with apricot preserves; Sunday was a scrambled egg or vanilla fat-free yogurt with banana slices, and a half a grapefruit with whole wheat toast, and so on. Every day, she ate her meal with a small glass of orange juice and a cup of decaffeinated coffee splashed with skim milk. She used a specific plate, bowl, utensil, and cup and saucer combination (some of which she'd held on to since my childhood, even though the finish had worn off) for each specific day of the week. If there was an interruption to her routine, my mother became anxious and cranky. She equated her set patterns with a sense of security, control, containment of chaos. "I'm a creature of comfort," she always said. "Like a cat."

"How're you feeling?" I asked.

"My body doesn't feel right," she said.

"What do you mean?" I asked.

"It's hard to explain," she said. "It just doesn't feel right."

I studied her, watched as she filled the teakettle with tap water and placed it on the electric stove. For a few moments, her breathing sounded labored, as if her lungs were rattling. She looked at me then. I tried to quickly shift my eyes so that she wouldn't think I was being intrusive, but it was too late, she'd seen me. Her breathing returned to normal.

"You're really worried about me," she said, smiling nervously, turning her gaze back to the breakfast preparations.

"Yes," I said. I could feel unconditional love between us. "I am."

"I'll be fine," she said, stepping from one side of the kitchen to the other to plug in the toaster oven. "It just takes me a while to get going in the morning."

"Can I help you with anything?" I asked.

"No," she said. "But after breakfast, will you come with me to buy the newspaper?" She purchased the *New York Times* every day, refusing home delivery.

"Why don't you let me drive?" I offered.

"Why?" she said. "I can drive."

I didn't want to tell her that I was afraid to be in the passenger seat with her at the wheel. Several years back, I sat beside her as she lost control of the car when we went over a patch of black ice. We were rounding a downhill curve beside the cemetery located at the exit of my mother's condo complex and I held my breath as the tombstones grew larger and larger through the windshield, as we went toward them in what felt like hair-raising slow motion. My mother regained steerage of the vehicle just before we hit a ditch beside the fence that divided the road from the first row of graves.

Now, I worried my mother might stop breathing and pass out while driving.

After breakfast, we got into her car just as the rain from the approaching hurricane, now downgraded to a tropical storm, was starting to blotch the pavement. I pulled the seatbelt across my body as my mother placed the key in the ignition switch, pausing for a moment before turning on the engine. I tried to ignore my fear that she might fall unconscious at the wheel, make my world go spinning. Part of me thought she wanted to die and take me with her. Part of me was willing. I thought perhaps that was why I was there: I didn't want her to go through death by herself. Looking back, I shudder at the way I was willing to put my own safety at risk, at how I so easily slipped into the old dynamic she'd placed me in when I was a girl: I was to sacrifice my well-being for my mother. Such were the terms of our love exchange.

Fortunately, we drove the five minutes to the shopping center without incident.

"There's the bank where I have my safety deposit box," my mother pointed to a short rectangular building on our right. "I've already shown Russell, but I wanted you to see it, too. That's where you'll go, if anything happens."

She meant if she died.

She drove around the curve in the parking lot, bringing us alongside a CVS. "I want to parallel park," she announced.

After she parked and we got out of the car, my mother walked around to the curb to admire her technique: "I haven't lost my touch," she said.

The rain was beginning to fall harder now, and my mother opened her umbrella and held it over both our heads.

"Maybe you should start heading back to Boston," my mother said as we walked the few steps to the CVS entranceway. "Before the weather gets too bad."

"I'll leave early this afternoon as I'd planned," I said. It was only mid-morning. Although I wanted to be back in my own surroundings, I didn't feel ready to leave my mother yet.

"Whatever you want," she said.

She purchased the *New York Times*, and then we were on our way back to the condo, traversing the winding hilly road of the complex. The rain had let up and my mother stopped the car at the top of a hill. "Maybe we could take a brief walk," she said. "I'd like to go to the brook."

The brook was a place where my mother liked to meditate. She hadn't been able to physically get herself there for over two weeks.

"Sure," I agreed.

We got out of the car and began to walk in the direction of the brook when my mother's breathing began to sound labored. She stopped to focus on her inhales and exhales. I felt my pulse quicken.

"Are you okay?" I asked.

"I just need to rest for a minute," she said. "I think it's anxiety."

"Okay," I said, standing beside her. "There's no rush, just take your time."

After a few breaths, she pushed on. Just ahead were the dense trees that lined the brook. I stopped at the curb, letting my mother go onward without me, her feet brushing through the wet, muddy grass.

"I'll wait here," I said, feeling as if I were giving my mother permission to go.

She charged ahead. When she reached the trees about thirty feet from where I stood, she paused and looked down where the brook was located, deep in the Earth's crevice. I'd stood beside her there once before, so that now I could imagine what she was doing even though her back was to me: She closed her eyes, letting the sound of the water washing the rock-filled path below fill her ears. She swept her arms above her head three times, bowing slightly as if in prayer.

Then she returned to me. "I feel a lot better now," she said.

She looked a lot better, too: There was color in her face, life in her body.

———

When we got back to her condo, she brought me into her bedroom, took a small bronze key from her pocketbook, and showed me how to get into her locked desk drawer, revealing the location of a gray lockbox for which there was a smaller second key and in which I'd find her "important papers, if something were to happen," she said. She'd shown me the location of her drawer periodically over the years of her good health but as an afterthought. Now, she conducted my orientation in great detail, as if it were a dress rehearsal.

She led me to the kitchen and showed me her address book, which she kept beside the phone. "Here are the important phone numbers." She pointed to the names of a few local friends and acquaintances: "Phyllis knows about the cemetery and the rabbi." What I wouldn't know until after her death was that my mother had already selected and paid for her cemetery plot. She continued, "Janice knows the people I'm friendly with at the synagogue."

She ran her finger down a list of women's names under the header "social action committee," a small group with whom she'd begun to gather monthly to perform Tzedakah, the Jewish tradition of community charity.

She asked if I wanted to have a copy of the information to take with me. I said yes. She handed me a pen and a piece of paper.

"I don't want an obituary in the newspaper," she said.

"You don't?" I asked.

"No," she shook her head.

"Why not?" A feeling of graveness came over me then, and I understood. "Because of Dad?"

Her eyes watered: She believed my father could hurt her even after her death.

"The people who care about me will know," she said, her lips quivering slightly before she breathed herself into a resolved stoicism, "and they will come."

In her next breath, she discussed her upcoming week's work schedule and her plans to enroll in a yoga class for the fall, as if her death weren't imminent.

She changed the subject again, investing her attention in the photos of her girlhood, which she kept in a box in her bedroom on top of my great-grandmother's small black wooden nightstand. She paged through her decades, asking if I'd remember the personal stories behind the images she shared. She reviewed the history of the framed artwork on her walls: She believed her late uncle had painted one piece; her younger sister had crafted another. I told her I'd remember, even though I didn't think I could. Everything was too much to hold.

———————————

The storm was drawing closer and I felt an urgent pull to return home. I hugged my mother goodbye.

"Thank you for visiting," she said. Her body felt warm and soft against me. "The best part was when you said you forgive me."

My words had reached her.

"I do," I said, rubbing her back with the palm of my hand. "I do."

"I love you very much," she said.

"I love you, too," I said.

She walked me to my car. In the misty air, beside my old Honda Civic, we embraced again.

I opened the door to my car, lowered myself into the driver's seat, and turned the key in the ignition. Then I got out of the car.

My mother looked surprised.

"One more hug," I said to her.

She smiled.

I drew her to me, held her. I didn't want to say goodbye, but I knew I truly had to now. "I love you very much," I repeated.

"I love you, too," she said.

Then I returned to my vehicle, shut the door, and secured my seatbelt. My mother stepped away, holding her umbrella over her head as I backed out of the parking spot. I placed the car gear stick in "drive." Pulling away, I waved. Looking in my rearview mirror, I watched my mother as she walked back to her condo. I watched as all I'd once yearned for her—and us—to fully be became smaller and smaller, until I turned a corner and my mother was gone.

When I reached the highway, the rain picked up with sudden force. I was surprised by how quickly the stronger waves of the storm moved in. The rain came down harder and harder, until the road was like an ocean of grief, disorienting me. On Connecticut's I-84, my car was like a ship at sea. I felt the vehicle hydroplaning. Visibility was only a few feet ahead. I was afraid I might get into an accident and die. It was too late to turn back, and I couldn't see the shoulder to pull off to wait things out.

My heart pounded and my throat began to constrict: I was having a panic attack. I turned on my emergency flashers and turned up the volume of the radio, blasting the only station I could access. "Come Sail Away," by Styx, began to play. With all my years of PTSD treatment, I knew that singing regulates breathing, which in turn helps the body and nervous system relax, so I sang along, loudly.

As the story within the song spilled from my lips, I thought about my mother and me. Tears drenched my cheeks and my nose began to run. I told myself I'd be okay; the rain would let up—it had to at some point.

I told myself to stay the course. Eventually I'd make it home, never more grateful for drier ground.

When I was growing up, my mother used to say that when she died she'd like to come back as a cat. When my grandmother passed, a gray Egyptian-looking feline began to regularly appear in our backyard, meeting our gaze. My mother thought it might be her mother visiting: "She had those cat eyes," my mother said, as if the cat were a comfort to her.

Like a cat, my mother prepared to die: She isolated herself, withdrew to a corner of the world. In the days following my visit, she didn't show up to her doctor's appointment and she didn't answer her phone. She only reached out after Russell and I were both contacted by her oncologist demanding to know where our mother was, and Russell and I couldn't reach her and decided we should send the police. My mother was home, and alive. She blamed the storm and subsequent down wires for her lack of landline phone communication; she had a cell phone but only turned it on for "emergencies."

She'd pass away a few days later. I was volunteering at the Animal Rescue League, trying to coax a frightened cat out from under his bed, where he'd burrowed himself inside his shelter cage, when I got the call from Aunt Nikki. My mother had checked herself into the hospital, her vitals were failing, I'd better come. My heart pounded, *no, no.* Adrenaline mopped my mouth. I grabbed my purse and ran.

On the T, en route to the garret, I made lists in my head: who to tell, what to bring. When the train finally arrived at Porter Square station, I rushed up the steep escalator and to the street, where my cell phone reception returned, and I called my friend Alison who lived nearby with her husband, five cats, and a Bichon. She arrived at my door shortly after I did. I gave her a set of my keys so she'd be able to come in and feed Hannah and Sam in my absence.

"Is there anything else I can do?" she asked.

All I could think was that nobody could do anything.

A quarter of the way into the four-hour drive to the hospital, I was delayed by a swarm of cars congesting the tollbooth that marked the line between I-90 and I-84. *Go, go*, I said half-aloud, gritting my teeth, trying to will the vehicles to clear my path. On the radio, Barry Manilow started singing "I Write the Songs." He was my mother's favorite singer and it'd been years since I'd heard him played on a mainstream station. I looked through the windshield at the sky where the clouds were like closed eyelids, the lashes spilling streaks of light. *You don't have to rush*, I thought I heard my mother whispering in my ear, *I'm already gone.*

According to the nurse, upon arrival at the emergency room my mother, drifting in and out of consciousness, reported that she'd felt a sense of doom for the past two days: "I know this is the end," my mother had told her, before she fell into permanent respiratory failure.

By the time I arrived at the ICU, my mother's cheeks and forehead were swollen from the ventilator, her blood pressure was destabilized, her eyes were closed, and her arms were swinging back and forth across the gurney, toward me, then away from me, as if her upper body were a pendulum on a grandfather clock, saying it was time.

Eighteen hours later, she died.

I stood beside her, watching the monitor as her blood pressure dropped lower and lower, holding her hand, feeling myself letting go of the possibility of ever having the mother I'd wanted and needed her to be.

Dream Lover

I DIDN'T DATE while my mother was dying, but that doesn't mean I didn't look.

He looked like he came out of a J. Crew catalogue. A single, dirty-blond, blue-eyed, chiseled-faced, fit man in his mid-thirties, Brad was a Phillips Academy and Princeton alumnus and nonprofit company vice president who sat at a table next to mine on Sunday mornings at the neighborhood café. His mother, a longtime volunteer with a suicide hotline, had died when he was in his twenties; he'd experienced the death of a loved one and therefore I assumed he held the same values I did on what was important and meaningful in love and life. His bio, coupled with his good looks and nice personality, made him my dream lover: I wanted him.

We introduced ourselves to each other when I was writing a book and he was answering what appeared from the expression on his face to be some very serious email, and he needed an outlet to plug in the power cord for his laptop; the nearest one was under my table.

"I think I used to see you at the Starbucks across the street," I said, which was an understatement. For a year, I'd ogled him from three window seats down, trying to think of an excuse to say hello. Then the Starbucks closed for renovations and I lamented that I'd never see him again. Then I went across the street to this café.

Brad smiled warmly. "Yeah, I remember you," he said.

He remembered me? I felt myself blush. "I'm Tracy," I said.

He put out his hand to shake mine. "Brad," he said. "Thanks for introducing yourself."

I thought he might like me.

For a year, every Sunday morning I went to the café and inevitably saw Brad sitting at a table, his gaze glued to his computer screen until he took the chance to look up, at me. Every Sunday morning I said hi, asking how his week had been. And every Sunday morning Brad smiled and asked me the same. Our conversations were brief—he always seemed intent on getting back to his work—but they were, I thought, deeper than superficial chitchat.

I never paid attention to the fact that he never asked me to join him.

When my mother died, Brad was one of the few peers I knew who understood what I was going through. Along with the long-ago loss of his mother, his father had recently passed. Talking with each other, we realized that he was going to be cleaning out his parents' house the same weekend I was going to be cleaning out my mother's condo. We'd both be doing it alone, together.

How morbidly romantic, I thought. I wondered if it was fate: Death was a tie to bind us.

I imagined asking him out, how he'd say yes. I imagined we'd date and, several months later, when my lease was up, I'd move out of the garret and Brad would move out of his place and we'd move in to a nice apartment together. A year after that, if things worked out, perhaps we'd get engaged, and then we'd get married. A couple years later, we'd have children. I daydreamed: It wasn't too late for me; I could still attain the kind of (love) life I wanted.

Though I'd made a lot of progress in my PTSD recovery, I was slipping back into an old habit: I was constructing a mirage, searching for a panacea, trying to force love to happen.

When I asked him out, I didn't think he'd say, "I think you're a very thoughtful person, but I don't think you're my type," or that he'd want to "just be friends," or that "we should have coffee sometime" or that every time after, when I'd walk into the café, he'd always be too busy with his laptop to "have coffee." I'd ponder over what it was about me that made me not his type; I'd consider that perhaps I'd come off as too tentative or too desperate to be attractive in the eyes of a guy I thought was "the whole package."

What I didn't consider was that perhaps he wasn't "the whole package."

What I didn't consider was that it wasn't just about me but about Brad, too, that he was flawed, just as I was, and that perhaps he wasn't available and not because he was taken (he wasn't—I saw he had an active profile on Match.com) but because he was always working on his laptop, a virtual curtain behind which he was hiding out from the world of relationships.

Once, a few months after I asked him out, I was walking down the street in my sexy white jeans, and I saw, in the distance, a man standing by his car, staring at me. He was looking at me in the way a man says "you're hot" with his eyes instead of his voice. As I got closer, I saw it was Brad. His gaze didn't match his stance about dating me. He said hello and mentioned he was meeting with a realtor: He was tired of renting and was considering buying a condo. Then he drove away.

Despite this encounter, our interactions at the café remained as they'd always been, until, at some point, Brad stopped coming. I figured he'd found a girlfriend and had no reason not to stay home in bed on Sunday mornings. Eventually, I moved to another part of town and frequented a different café, one closer to where I lived.

For a long while, I forgot about him.

———

A few years into the future, I'd get curious and Google him, thinking I might find a wedding announcement. Instead, I'd find his obituary.

Brad had died of brain cancer, which the obituary stated he'd battled for four years. Four years before his death was around the time we'd first introduced ourselves to each other.

My friends would suggest that Brad hadn't wanted to pursue a relationship with me not because he didn't care for me but because he was trying to protect me. That may or may not have been true. But what is true is that, when I knew him, I made many assumptions, rooted in my low self-esteem.

You know that saying about how people come into your life for a reason, a season, or a lifetime? I believe Brad came into my life for a reason: to mirror my idea of a dream partner, and to bring my frame of reference beyond my self-critical thinking. Brad wouldn't be my future boyfriend or husband, but he taught me to believe that such a person existed. And that person wasn't perfect: He was *real*.

Life is short and doesn't always turn out the way we want or plan. I think Brad would agree. We can't always change our circumstances, but we can honor the path we're on. Sometimes, when we meet a potential partner, we might just be on mismatched timelines—one of us might not be able to be in a relationship at that very moment, for whatever reason. It's sad but it's true: A rejection may have nothing at all to do with you, and everything to do with the other person.

Sometimes, feeling discouraged about finding the love of my life, I'd visit that old café and catch myself, for an instant, looking for Brad. I'd know he was gone, but the gift of him would always remain.

The Power of Love

SLOWLY BUT SURELY, I was moving onward.

That morning, the road was dark. No highway lights arched overhead to illuminate my path, to distinguish between ground and sky. It was as if I was driving through a black hole. Every so often another vehicle passed—for a moment, I was no longer alone—and I followed the taillights until their blood-shot glow dimmed and disappeared into the oblivion ahead.

Disoriented, I turned on the high beams of my now twelve-year-old Honda Civic, which allowed me to see only a few hundred feet ahead. My eyes were fixed on where the road curved and appeared to end.

I'd left my apartment at 5 a.m., in darkness, to drive to my mother's condo in New York, where I was going to clean her home into a state of "sale-able" condition and meet with a realtor to put the property on the market. Russell had gone two weeks earlier to sell our mother's car; however, at the time, he couldn't bear to be inside her condo but briefly.

This was my charge.

All along the solitary route, I felt a familiar and persistent void: the absence of a partner. I'd asked my closest friend Lisa to come with me, but she declined. Her mother was recently diagnosed with the same cancer my mother had, and she simply couldn't tolerate the emotional journey. I understood. I didn't think I could do it myself.

I drove onward, waiting for the sun to rise, telling myself night would turn to day—*this is earth science, this is a given*—that darkness would give way to light, though it wasn't until I crossed the Connecticut border that, far off on the horizon, I glimpsed the beginning of dawn.

When I arrived at my mother's condo complex, I parked the car in her empty spot and shook the stiffness from my legs as I climbed the cement steps that led to a narrow tree-lined tar-paved path, which curved and ended at my mother's front door. There, I stood on her old welcome mat, taking in the stillness that surrounded me. The one-syllable chirp of a bird intermittently pierced the silence.

I looked to the peephole, considering what it would feel like to be on the other side, inside. With my eyes, I traced the upper right corner of the door-frame down a few inches to the mezuzah, which my mother once nailed securely at its required customary slant. The casing was weathered by time.

I half-expected my mother to open the door to greet me. Then I reminded myself, *she's dead.* I took her key from my purse, unlocked the door, and went in.

The mustiness of my late grandmother's old red sofa chairs made me catch my breath. My grandmother had suffered terrible psoriasis and her skin, which held a peculiar odor (a combination of medicinal cream and dead epidermis), sloughed off translucent brittle patches, showering a trail wherever she went. When my grandmother died, when I was twelve, my mother held on to the cluster of three red sofa chairs that fit together in a semi-circle, and when she sold our house and moved to the condo she brought them with her. When Russell or I visited, we asked her to clean the chairs to get rid of the smell, and she promised, however my grandmother's scent remained. Although my mother said she'd replace the set with a pullout couch—not because of the odor but because my brother and I didn't have a place to sleep—she never followed through.

The sofa chairs stood in my mother's living room, a mausoleum where the remnants of my childhood remained. Photographs of family affairs—Bar and Bat Mitzvahs, high school and college graduations, reunions—posed on the tops of two white-painted bookcases as well as above the fireplace, which my mother, out of fear, never lit.

The window shades were drawn, as she'd left them.

I turned to the short hall, making my way toward my mother's bedroom on the left and the bathroom on the right, next to the washer and dryer where I'd stood beside my mother as she sorted her laundry the day I disclosed the abuse.

I tried not to think about memories: I didn't want to get stuck in them. I had a task to complete.

———————

I began to empty my mother's most personal spaces: the medicine cabinet with the Coumadin, packages of syringes, and Crest white strips; the sock drawer, where I found an envelope filled with a handful of my mother's hair, which she'd kept after losing it during chemotherapy; and the underwear drawer where, under a pile of neatly stacked briefs, I uncovered a folded Wonder bra with the tags still attached.

My mother's personal effects were pristinely neat. She economized space, but the more I sifted through, took in, and disposed of the items of her intimate life, those things she shared with no one, the more there appeared to be.

I had to go through her life in order to discard it.

I collated her casual and professional clothing, taking in the patterns of her days: fifty-six shirts, thirty-nine blouses, twenty-five sweaters, eight sweater jackets, ten pairs of shorts, fifteen casual pants, four skirts, four pairs of casual gloves, three pairs of dress gloves, five scarves with a pin set, seven pairs of casual shoes, six pairs of dress shoes/heels, ten warm-up suits, twelve dress suits, four pairs of slacks, three lightweight jackets, one wool winter coat, one rain-coat, three casual coats, two blankets, ten blazer jackets, and one belt.

I organized the wardrobe into piles on my mother's queen-sized bed, which she'd taken the time to make before she left to check herself into the emergency room the day before she died. She'd tucked the sheets into tight hospital corners, smoothing out the wrinkles before covering it all with her emerald green bedspread patterned with pink roses.

In a cubby in her closet, I came upon my mother's work portfolio, which was maroon leather, worn and hardened by time and secured by a gold-colored metal clasp that I opened by pressing my thumb down on its tiny latch. Inside, I found a master copy editor's style sheet and general house style sheet, which my mother had created when she became the head copy editor at the book publisher. The style sheets were lengthy and detailed, noting the rules: when to use capital letters, when to use lowercase, when to spell out numbers, how to abbreviate, when to use the em-dash, when to use the en-dash, and the list went on.

Paging through her portfolio, I was reminded of the way she valued accuracy. There were conversion tables used so often the paper was frayed and limp—feet to meters, inches to millimeters, degrees Celsius to degrees Fahrenheit, grams to avoirdupois ounces, grams to avoirdupois kilograms, metric conversion quarts to liters, kilometers to miles and yards. There was a list of state abbreviations, and a style sheet for a series of pet manuals with the addendum "weight measurements decimal ok, use common fractions for linear and liquid measurements" cursively written in red ballpoint ink.

In a side pocket was a monogrammed planner in which she kept an index card with a typewritten quote from David Leavitt's novel, *The Lost Language of Cranes*: "She was a copy editor, possessed of the rare capacity to sit all day in a small cubicle, like a monk in a cell, and read with an almost penitential rigor."

That was her talisman, though to me it appeared to be her epitaph.

My mother's portfolio reflected, with the sharpest clarity, her supreme attention to detail. Her greatest, most prioritized value and skill was spotting and fixing mistakes, what she described on her resumé as "maintaining the integrity of the work." No improper detail got past her eagle eyes, and yet, when I was growing up, she "let stand" the most overarching errancy of all: the abusive home in which we lived, a realm ruled by the man who marred my childhood and terrorized her married life.

My mother's middle desk drawer held several pens and pencils, and blank square and rectangular post-it notes, and an appointment calendar, and a miniature green Mead notebook in which she kept recorded logs of her interactions with my father: how he'd accused her of monopolizing my time and taking me away from him—"I'll remember this and get you back," he said; how, when she rented a car to take me to my two-day college orientation, he said, "How much are you soaking me for this time? You only put your hands down my pockets for money"; and how, when she didn't respond, he called her "deaf and dumb":

Sun. Nov 1, 1992, 4 p.m.

I am downstairs ironing. (Earlier in the afternoon I had walked down the street to meet Nikki, who was to pick me up at 12:30. I didn't want her to run into [my husband], who was getting ready to go out. When I got to the corner of [our street], neighbor Arielle Sawyer was outside bagging leaves. She saw me standing there and asked, "Is everything alright?" I said, "Yes." We spoke a bit about the children. I told her Russell had taken the car and I was without one for the day. Then [my husband] pulled up in his car, rolled down the window and called out, "Do you have your key?" I was standing there with my handbag. I nodded "yes." He still stood, so Arielle went over to the car and he just said he wanted to make sure I wasn't locked out. Then he sped off. I left Arielle, walked back to the house, and waited for Nikki.)

He says, "You know, I just wanted to make sure you had your keys. Next time I'll leave you stranded outside until your nipples freeze off. I don't know what you've been telling the neighbors, but I think it's really uncool. Do you have anything to say?"

I say, "Nope."

He storms upstairs, only to return a few minutes later.

He says, "And another thing, next time you need extra money for a doctor's appointment (I went for my mammography on Fri and paid $115, which left only $150 in checking after he deposited $100 on Thurs.) tell me ahead of time. It's bad enough you're skimming money off the grocery bill. That's all you know is to put your hand in my pocket. You don't reach for anything else, just my money."

I say, "There's supposed to be $1,000 put in the account each month." (He only put in $600, + $200, + $100—doling it out so I feel strapped.)

He says, "I don't know where you got that amount. I put in what's needed."

He storms back upstairs.

Reading my mother's account, I saw my father from her point of view, how she lived under the reign of abuse. I wondered if she had recorded their interactions because she was afraid he might kill her. Her fear was palpable on the page.

After several blank pages noting the end of her record of my father's behavior, amidst her documentation of my father's monthly alimony payments, my mother wrote drafts of a dating ad:

Warm, intelligent ~~woman~~ blue-eyed blonde seeks caring, secure ~~middle-age man~~ (45-55) professional to share life's more subtle moments.

Warm, ~~sensitive~~ intelligent woman ~~seeking~~ seeks caring, secure middle-age man to share life's ~~subtler~~ more subtle moments.

comfortable
~~share~~ enjoy
get more from life
happy way

I didn't know if my mother ever posted her ad, but despite her experiences with my father I knew that for a time after the divorce she'd wanted to find a partner. I recalled how she sometimes mentioned to me that she'd like to have a companion. Her desire had given me hope. However, as the years went by, as she became more and more austere, she let go of the idea.

———

My mother's friend Phyllis offered to help me.

"I once accompanied a friend on a staging excursion," Phyllis explained when she arrived, walking into my mother's bedroom, her eyes landing on my mother's desk, the top of which I'd cleared. She bent down to the floor and pointed underneath.

"That needs to be cleaned up," she said. I saw the blood flowing to her head, reddening her face.

I didn't know what Phyllis saw. All I knew was that I didn't want to clean up more of my mother's things.

I leaned over. "There's nothing valuable left," I said. "I think I should wait until after the realtor takes a look. He'll know how things should be prepared."

But Phyllis wasn't listening. She was reaching deep under my mother's desk as if to begin an excavation. I got down beside her and saw a shelf overflowing with loose folders above a row of spiral notebooks. I felt my pulse pound across my forehead.

"These things should be filed neatly in boxes," Phyllis said as she retrieved a handful, "which you can stack on the floor of the closet."

Stretching my arm beneath the desk, I wrapped my fingers around a couple of notebooks and pulled them toward me, quickly flipping through pages of my mother's writing from the 1980s, drafts of poetry and prose she'd crafted in her mid-to-late thirties, when she was my age.

"Are these important?" Phyllis pushed a few folders at me. Before I could answer, she handed me more. "What are these?" She placed folder after folder in my hands. "And these?" I saw an overstuffed folder from my college freshman orientation. Inside were several envelopes with my younger handwriting on them.

The idea sunk in: My mother had held on to my letters.

My mother had also held on to contentious emails between us from the years following my PTSD diagnosis. She'd written notes in the margins, things she'd wanted to say to me but never did. Attached to the top of one printout was a rectangular pale-yellow post-it note on which my mother drew two columns. She labeled one column "T doesn't want," and, underneath it, she listed things that I'd said bothered me about her behavior: *be anxious, to hear my problems, to get sick (can't sleep) over her [T's] problems, to ask her [T] for support, me to hide things.* She labeled the other column "T wants" and enumerated what she believed I was asking of her: *calm/support, listen to her problems, provide advice/*

solutions (detach myself emotionally), keep my needs to myself (or confide in a friend), let her know what's happening (but keep low-key—no stress on her part), to be closer to me.

While some of what my mother noted wasn't entirely accurate from my perspective, my attention got stuck on the final phrase, *to be closer to me.* Even though my ("T's") wish appeared last in the list, it wasn't inconsequential. It was unmistakable, in black and white: My mother had taken in that I'd wanted to be closer to her.

The truth was there in indelible ink.

The day my mother died, after I left the hospital with Russell and Aunt Nikki and her husband, Charlie, who'd driven up to New York from where they lived in North Carolina, we went back to my mother's condo and I retrieved my mother's lockbox from her bedroom, as per her instructions. Inside, amidst her legal and financial documents, was a sealed envelope with my name on it. It was a Hallmark "Between You and Me" card. On the cover was a printed message: *I believe in you . . . in your spirit, your goodness, in the way that you face each day with a commitment to your life and the things that really matter. I believe in the decisions you make, in the careful consideration you give each challenge, in the perseverance you've shown when others might have given up. I believe that you possess an extraordinary strength and endless reserve of resilience—even more than you realize.* Inside the card, the message continued: *You are a person of enormous courage, someone truly special in this world, a rare and beautiful gift to all of us . . . And I hope you'll never forget that I believe in you!* In a blank space, using blue ballpoint ink, my mother penned her own thoughts:

Your inner beauty and delightful ways have brought me much joy over the years. I am so proud of you, as my daughter. Thank you for being you. I wish you peace, happiness, and light, always, for you have given so much of yourself. Remember, I am close by always, in your thoughts and heart. I love you very much—Mom

At first I didn't know if I could trust such loving words, the opposite of my mother's harsh and negative messages to me over the years. But, reading the notes my mother secretly kept, I came to believe that what she'd written in the card was her true voice, her essence, unencumbered by the defenses that had held her back, out of reach, when she was alive.

Now, I noticed a sliver of newsprint poking out of a thick manila folder that Phyllis had handed me. I caught the word "abuse" in a headline. My body grew hot.

I opened the folder. Inside were articles on child sexual abuse, highlighted and underlined in many places by my mother as if she'd been annotating them to study and master, just as she might have assembled the details of a style manual. There were loose legal pad pages full of her handwriting outlining facts from books about the mother's role in father-daughter incest, the perpetrator's personality, denial, family system theory, the adult child coping with PTSD, and the path to heal from life-altering trauma.

From the dates of the more than two-dozen newspaper articles, I deduced that my mother had penned her notes and collected clippings over the course of seven years, beginning a year after I'd disclosed the abuse to her and ending the year of her cancer diagnosis. Newspaper headlines included "Abuse Charges Against a Coach Now Dead," "Teacher Admits Molesting Pupils," "Unsafe at Any Age," "Why We Shouldn't Be Surprised by the Jackson Verdict," "The Incest Loophole," and "The Secret Lives of Just About Everybody."

I imagined my mother's face as she came upon these stories, with their sordid details. In her living room, in the evening after a long day of work or on the weekend, she sat with the soft white lamplight shining down on the newspaper, which she held open in front of her in the manner she always had, with one side grasped in each hand so that the publication surrounded her entire upper body like armor.

Her blue eyes were round as full moons behind her glasses, and as she came upon something in particular, her thin and pale blonde eyebrows rose. She stood and carried the newspaper into the kitchen, where she removed from the drawer a pair of scissors she'd owned since I was in elementary school. She neatly cut out an article. With a black ballpoint pen, she labeled its date of publication, if such data was not printed in the portion she'd detached. She marked lines and paragraphs, underscoring what was most important. Sometimes, she used a yellow highlighter.

In such a manner, day after day, year after year, my mother accrued these articles as if they were an ever-growing stockpile of evidence pointing to who did what to whom, and where, and when. Looking to the printed word, she inquired into how and why.

In the years after my disclosure, I'd asked my mother many times to talk openly about what had happened in our family, about how it still affected me, us, but she refused. "I won't be able to function," she repeated.

Case closed. Discussion over.

During the broom sweep of the property, I learned that my mother had begun to write again. Within a clear plastic sleeve was a poem my mother had composed when I was thirty-four. Titling the piece "Hindsight," she expressed her wish to go back to my childhood to save me from the abuse, and her desire, in my adulthood, to help me heal.

The truth was in my hands. In secret, my mother had gone to great lengths to grapple with a life-changing mistake. In private, she'd closely examined the details, incidents she could not go back in time to change, to rectify. She tried to wrap her mind around the whole terrible story.

My mother was unable to speak the truth aloud, to openly utter the words, or to enact her deepest intentions, but she left behind her organized collection of facts and thoughts and feelings for me to discover, to know, to say, *I see, I hear, I know.*

I love you, I'm sorry.

CHAPTER 10
YOU GOTTA BELIEVE

Dear Future Life Partner,

After my mother's death, I spent a year settling her affairs while trying to cope with my grief. My mother had named Russell and me co-executors of her will. As we worked together, we often came into conflict, because of our opposing styles of handling stress. In the process, we grew to understand each other and the effects our upbringing had had on both of us as individuals. As time went on, our relationship improved and we became closer as siblings.

For a while, I found it difficult to cultivate a mindset for socializing—some days I could barely focus on one simple task without feeling completely overwhelmed. But I did put myself back in the ring. I began to date again, with a new attitude: carpe diem. Without my mother harping critically about my choices, I felt less restricted, free. Dealing with her passing helped me commit to seeking out what I valued and wanted most: genuine, close, lasting relationships.

I began to consider that my life turning out differently than the way I'd once planned might not be the end of the world, but the very beginning.

———

Where were you during these years? What was your life like? Were you engaged or married, or single, or happy? What did you want, and what or whom did you have?

Did you go on date after date, as I did, wondering if you'd ever find me? Or did the thought of me never occur to you, until the day we met?

For years, I judged myself for my flaws and my fears, for everything I didn't do, for the voice inside that shut me down, keeping me from finding you. But eventually

I came to believe that I'd done all that I could. For so long, I'd tried to make my life happen instead of allowing it to unfold. I was afraid that if I let go of trying to control everything, I'd find out that I didn't have a future. But the reality was, I did.

The past was not a determinant of the destiny of my love life. Focusing on the possibilities of the present, I started to have confidence that things would naturally work out.

My Dating Life Is Not Doomed

SOMETIMES, JUST WHEN we reach a landing in life, the universe throws us a little challenge, a tenacity test of sorts. Just when I thought I'd put my past behind me, just as I was starting to have real hope for my future, I came up against the doubts of others.

"Don't you understand that a man isn't going to be able to handle your history?" Serena asked.

There'd been turnover in my coed relationship therapy group. The men who'd supported me previously were no longer members. The four other current group members—two men and two women—agreed with Serena, who believed I was going to be rejected by every man I tried to date, because I was an incest survivor. The fact that I was still single at thirty-nine was proof, they said.

"When I go on a date," Serena continued, "I don't announce that I have daddy issues. I let the guy get to know me first."

She was making a point regarding my online presence. My dating profile said nothing about my history, and I didn't announce it on my dates. But I'd published essays about grappling with and overcoming my past, and some of those essays were in high profile publications that were accessible online. A potential boyfriend could Google my name and read all about it. The group saw my past as a "Scarlet A," and my publications as a destructive megaphone that announced my "sullied" status before I ever met my future life partner in person.

The group leader, Tara, a middle-aged clinical social worker, concurred: "You should remove your essays from the web so that it's not searchable. I think you need to have control over how and when men find out about your history."

I agreed that it was beneficial to have control over self-disclosure, but I wasn't ashamed of my publications, or the past I'd worked hard to transcend. In fact, I was proud of the work I'd done. Even if removing my essays were possible, I didn't understand why, in order to become an acceptable girlfriend or acquire a life partner, I had to suppress something vital about myself: the fact that I'm a writer.

"I wouldn't tell the guy you're a writer," said Jamie, a group member who'd just ended a two-year relationship. "Just say you're a teacher and leave it at that."

"At least withhold your last name," said Bill.

My dating life would otherwise be doomed: No man would want to be in a relationship with me, the group decreed.

I wondered, how long did they think I could keep basic details, such as my full name, from a potential boyfriend? Still, the group mentality was hard for me to rebuff. I'd spent so much of my life questioning myself. Now, outnumbered, I began to lose the self-confidence and self-worth I'd worked so hard to build.

I knew this: Years before I'd published anything, I dated from a place of fear. Before my PTSD diagnosis, it was fear of sexual assault; after my PTSD diagnosis, it was fear of rejection. Believing the mere knowledge of the events of my past was detrimental to a potential relationship, I went on dates worried about the moment a man would find out the one fact I imagined would be more of a deal breaker than infidelity or a drug habit or an STD: incest. I saw myself as damaged goods. I worked hard to keep conversations away from the topics of family and parents and where I grew up, anything that could potentially reveal my truth. In doing that, however, I wasn't being myself. I presented myself in a way that wasn't real. Actively avoiding certain topics squelched my personality, which cut my chance of developing an authentic connection.

I was beyond that now.

I didn't feel the need to announce to anyone I just met—a potential boyfriend, neighbor, colleague, whomever—something so personal. But, I told the group, I couldn't stop people from asking questions or going online and searching for information. "And I'm not afraid if they do," I said.

"That's a mistake," Serena said.

I disagreed. I no longer feared someone knowing the truth, and so I didn't understand why the group did. Sure, I had regrets about the way I'd coped during my young adulthood, but that was how I'd survived until I was able to deal with my problems. How did this make me less of a catch?

Despite my group's warnings, I continued to go out—with men I discovered were still married, despite their profiles claiming they were divorced; with men who lied about their age; with a man who told me online that he was a Harvard fellow and then disclosed on our date that that wasn't exactly true; with a man who lived with five roommates and couldn't hold down a job and just wanted a warm body.

None of these men wanted me. But I didn't want them either.

We all have problems. Some of us suffer from depression or anxiety, or we're commitment-phobic or controlling, or we have issues surrounding intimacy or anger or body image or self-esteem. We all have histories, and we're all shaped by life experiences. None of us is immune to baggage. We all have the choice to face it, or not.

Although we may not speak of our personal difficulties on first or second or even third dates, I know from experience that they announce themselves through our body language, our behaviors, our words, our decisions to stay or leave or drink or text or call or have sex or whatever it is we end up doing or not doing. Serena, for example, was terribly anxious about a man leaving her in the way her father had left her when she was a child, a painful experience of abandonment that she couldn't seem to let go of; she frequently got so drunk on dates that she blacked out and didn't recall how she got home. But she didn't see her unresolved "daddy issues" as a problem in her dating life. She avoided addressing her past. Instead, she pointed to my history as the thing that was taboo.

We unconsciously reveal and reenact what we don't mindfully acknowledge.

———————

We pick up cues and draw conclusions about each other.

"I feel like I know you!" Kristoff exclaimed when we met for the first time. Drinking espresso, he explained he'd read several of my essays, which he'd found online by searching on Google for my first name, "writer," and "Boston," terms from my dating profile.

Kristoff didn't reject me because of my history.

When he proclaimed that he felt he knew me because he'd read my essays, at first I was relieved, because I no longer had to wonder about what his reaction would be to finding out about my past. But by our second date I was irritated, because he was making incorrect assumptions about who I was as a person, based upon what he'd read.

When I decided to stop seeing him because, among other reasons, he was living with two women and was obsessed with thinness and seemed, in our interactions, to be looking for a mother rather than a partner, he sent me a note trying to convince me that he was my match: "Having read that you are a victim of familial sexual abuse, I thought that my gentle and nurturing disposition might be an okay fit for you, that being the archetypal caretaker and someone who treads very gently around personal emotional issues might complement your personality."

I wasn't looking for a caretaker; I was looking for a partner.

Yes, I *was* a victim—during my childhood. I wasn't one in the present, nor was I a china doll. While I appreciated sensitivity and compassion, Kristoff wasn't seeing me as separate from my past. I suspected that was because he wasn't seeing himself as separate from his own.

Although I understood how Kristoff could easily think he knew me from reading my essays, he really didn't know me. The online presence is a persona, at its worst misleading, and at its best limited, incomplete. It doesn't capture the multidimensional person who exists in "real" life.

"I am not my essays," I told Kristoff. "That's why I thought we were going out, so that you could get to know me, and I could get to know you."

———

Was my dating life doomed? Did I understand that a man wasn't going to be able to handle my history? I no longer presumed anything about a man until I got to know him.

Ultimately, I believe it isn't about whether a man is able to handle my history; it's about the fact that *I* am able to handle my history. It's my history, after all. Only in taking responsibility for our issues and working through our pasts can any of us truly be available to fully be with others. And I hope that for my future life partner, that's what counts.

Eventually, I left the therapy group, because I found the ongoing conversation to be diminishing, at times bullying. I wasn't expecting affirmations or coddling, but I was looking for respect, and growth. There comes a point in life when you stop taking as the truth what others say or judge about you and your ability to be in relationships. While it was hard to shut off the voices of naysayers and critics, I knew myself best.

Tara, the leader, tried to convince me to stay in the group. She said I wouldn't find better circumstances elsewhere.

That was the lie my parents had fed me for decades.

As I was on my way out the door, Tara offered one last thought: "I think Serena and the others are afraid of real intimacy. You're not. For what it's worth."

I took note: Contrary to what I'd expected, my ability and desire for intimacy had caused the end of my relationship with the group, rather than a deeper bond. It wasn't a healthy situation. I could've stayed, as many people do in relationships that aren't working. Instead, I decided to cut my losses, to move on, to find what—and whom—I was looking for, and not look back.

What's Love Got to Do With It?

SOMETIMES LOVE HAS nothing to do with it—dating is just exhaustingly absurd.

Patience and perseverance are imperative. So is levity. After years of trying to find "Mr. Right," I came to understand the importance of taking some time to laugh about the process, especially when things went awry.

He practically had an orgasm at the table while talking about caramelizing onions. He said he loves to put scallions on his pasta, and that he taught himself a secret: You can cut your scallions down to the white part and put them in a glass of water and they'll regrow, up to three times. He told me he just turned forty-five and how difficult online dating is. Before we even ordered dinner at the Thai restaurant where we met for our first date, he suggested I move in with him in his condo in Brookline so that I wouldn't have to continue paying my high rent. He told me his dying father wants him to have children RIGHT NOW. He brought up the importance of Judaism and we argued over his belief that I'd be "watering down the species" by marrying a non-Jew even if the non-Jew would allow me to raise my kids Jewish. He asked what I like to do in my free time. I told him I like to hike, bike, and kayak. He replied, "What's a kayak?" Yes, he has a college degree and no, he's not an alien. I asked if he likes pets. He said he wants to own three to five dogs. I said I have two cats. He said he hopes this isn't a deal breaker but he's deathly allergic.

Oh, really? Darn.

I used to think that one miraculous day my dating life would suddenly change for the better. I went on each of my dates wondering if that moment had finally come. In each man I met, my heart eagerly searched for you, my life partner: "Are you him?" Well? I was growing tired of my dire and reflexive internal question, and the way I'd quickly find out, time and time again, that the answer was no.

"Desperation," Dr. Ross labeled my approach. "Grasping at something never works." He likened the issue to befriending a cat: Ever try to insist that a cat cuddle with you? It never works. But if you remain open, an interested cat comes to you, head butts your arm or leg, and takes a seat.

I'd learn, slower than I wished, to discern the difference between "grasping"— my attempt to gain control over the uncontrollable—and "trying," putting myself out there in an open way, without needing a partner to make me feel fulfilled. I clutched onto the former vibe until I grew tired of its burdensome weight. Only then did I put down my sense of expectation. Only then was I truly available for a real, satisfying connection.

Of course, that doesn't mean that you instantly appeared.

———————

He asked to meet for "a coffee date." At the café, he walked me over to the water fountain. He handed me a cup.

That was the date.

He was a hot ginger-haired chef with an advanced degree.

We met at a mandatory three-hour unemployment recipient meeting at Career Source in Cambridge. We were paired for a mock informational interview, an exercise meant to help unemployment recipients successfully reenter the workforce. Sitting beside each other, we shared our job losses, our struggles, our goals, and our wish for the meeting to conclude sooner rather than later.

We bantered. We flirted.

When we were finally dismissed, I raced out of the room and down the stairs.

"What, do you have a hot date or something?" the hot ginger-haired chef said, running after me, his voice echoing in the stairwell.

"Maybe," I said.

He chuckled.

What I had was a therapy appointment. I was going to be late.

I left the hot ginger-haired chef behind and dashed to my car. I shut the door, threw my purse onto the floor, and turned the key in the ignition.

On my way to the parking lot exit, I passed him.

Spontaneity struck. I stopped my car. I backed it up. I rolled down my window and handed him a piece of paper with my email address: "Write me," I said.

He took my info, and grinned.

I thought that maybe losing my job might have a silver lining after all. Maybe my misfortune wasn't an event marked by futility but one that had happened for a productive reason: meeting Mr. Right.

Twenty-four hours later, I found out that the hot chef was not Mr. Right when he sent me a photo of himself holding an Uzi.

He had a gun fetish.

And that was the end of that.

———————

Some dating stories aren't all that funny, in the moment. But after some time has passed, just when you least expect it, the cosmos delivers a twist, a point of cathartic relief.

His name was Jonathan. He was a professor, a rather serious-looking one, tall and fit as a basketball player, dark-haired and distinguished like a Disney prince. He was late thirty-something, though he looked mid-forty-something. He didn't have a beard or mustache, but he wasn't clean-shaven either. He wore a blazer and tie, and expensive shoes. He adjusted and readjusted the strap of his camel brown leather messenger bag, which he slung over his shoulder while he stood in the hallway before the start of class, keeping his eyes glued to his cell phone as he made rhythmical scrolling motions on the screen with his thumb, as if he were looking at a very important newsfeed or email, or pictures of his dog, a Doberman Pinscher. He appeared uneasy amidst the socializing students, and more comfortable at the front of the classroom, standing behind a lecture podium, in his role as an academic.

When I first met him, I wondered what he'd look like if he smiled.

The clunky gray university building where we taught was once a department store, its entranceway fashioned with a glass overhang shaped like the sun, with off-white opaque rays fanning outward. An American flag billowed from the rooftop. Muzak piped through the hallways of the first floor, where the university's central mailroom, bookstore, an ATM machine, bubble tea bar, a ramen noodle lunch counter, and a coffee café were located. Classrooms were situated on the second and third floors, where the interior department store layout didn't quite fit the institutional setting.

I introduced myself one day when I needed an eraser.

"Hi," I said, entering his room, which was located next door to mine, before class began.

When he looked at me I felt my cheeks get warm.

"Would you happen to have an extra eraser I could borrow?" I asked. "My classroom seems to be without one."

Jonathan glanced at the chalkboard. There was one eraser.

"Oh, you only have one," I said. "Never mind then." I turned to leave.

"Wait," Jonathan said, reaching for the eraser. "I don't need it."

"I guess you don't teach English composition then," I said.

"No," Jonathan said. He taught astronomy.

"I'm new here," I said. "I didn't realize I had to bring my own eraser to class."

He grinned in disgruntled commiseration, his brown eyes shining.

Every Monday and Wednesday in the hallway, during the minutes before the start of class, we griped about our adjunct professor life. I talked about losing my full-time job and Jonathan shared his five-year plight for the elusive tenure-track position. As an adjunct, he taught twenty classes a year at three different universities in order to earn a decent living.

"What?" I said, flabbergasted. I'd never taught more than eight classes a year, and that amount was grueling. A standard full-time faculty load was six per year, five at the tenure-track level, and generally three at full professor status. "How are you functioning?"

"You'd be surprised what you can get used to," Jonathan said. "The problem with teaching so many classes is I have no time to do my research."

Or date? I thought. I wondered if he was single, straight or gay. I leaned over to grab something in my bag, catching myself employing a quintessential flirty woman move. Did he check out my breasts? I didn't have the guts to look.

Later, I was in the middle of teaching a lesson on introductory paragraphs when I saw Jonathan, from the corner of my eye, tentatively entering my classroom.

"Would you have a piece of chalk I could borrow?" he asked rather sheepishly.

"Sure," I said, taking two pieces from the chalkboard and placing them in his palm. "Here you go." I felt the softness of his hand and electricity dancing on the tips of my fingers as they touched his skin.

I hoped my students didn't see me blush.

Over the course of the semester, we discussed how much less stressed we'd be if we didn't have to run around town to get to our second or third jobs on time, if we didn't have to be beggars when it came to wages and job security, if we didn't spend our Friday nights alone, writing job applications. Yes, it seemed, he was single. Together, we dreamed about how wonderful it would be to have one substantial gig, a stable place to land, a place where we'd belong.

Misery loves company, but I thought Jonathan and I had more going for us than that. He showed me photos of his dog, Abby—by this time, I'd worked through my fear of dogs in therapy and had actually grown quite fond of them, training them at the Animal Rescue League during my volunteer shift, though the thought of a Doberman did give me pause. I showed Jonathan a photo of my cats. I secretly fantasized about how we'd fall in love and move in together so that we could afford our rent. Then we'd both get hired at the same university for tenure-track positions. Then we'd get married and have kids.

Stop it, I told myself, *stop it*: How many times would I go down this road, getting ahead of myself, being unrealistic? I was setting myself up for royal disappointment. We hadn't even gone out on a date.

When I asked Jonathan if he'd like to meet up for coffee he said yes, but we never did because he was always running from class to another job at another university, and he wasn't free on weekends because he was either grading or jet-setting off to Miami to visit friends and play golf.

Mid-semester, in the hallway before class, he told me he'd just checked his email on his phone and received word that he was losing his job at another university where he'd been teaching as an adjunct for several years. This kind of termination was a common phenomenon for adjuncts, particularly once they met a particular college's pay ceiling. How was he to perform in the classroom after getting news like that?

"I'm sorry," I said. He looked devastated.

Later, I sent him an email: "I'd love to take your mind off it all for an hour or two. Do you have a favorite pub with a dartboard or coffee place? How about we take a break in the grading action this weekend and meet up for pizza and beer (though I dislike beer so I'll be the one having the wine cooler or nonalcoholic drink), and a vent-fest with mandatory laughs included, or Sunday brunch or a run around the Charles or something else of your choice. You name it."

He didn't respond. I felt annoyed at myself for possibly coming on too strong.

When I saw him before our next class, he thanked me for my email. He said he was sorry he hadn't replied. He'd been busy.

"We should have coffee one of these days," he said.

But then he was always busy. A few weeks later I casually said, "How about coffee next Monday after class?" But he was too busy again—he had to run off to another class, or home to walk Abby.

He was a workaholic: He never had time for anything personal.

On the last day of the semester, I decided to take a risk. I didn't want to wonder "what if." Not wanting to face rejection in person, I confessed my feelings for him via email:

Jonathan,

I've really enjoyed our before-class chats this term. I confess that our banter was, some days, my only incentive for going to work. I have no idea if you're single or in a relationship with someone, or if work is your main priority, but if you'd be interested in getting to know each other outside of the academic setting, let me know. I have a feeling, given your lack of a "yes" to my previous invitations etc, that you probably don't have the same feelings towards me as I've developed for you, and no worries if that is the case. Such is life! But I didn't want to regret not saying something.

Tracy

He didn't respond via email. He came to my classroom, walking in just after my students left.

"I got your note," he said.

"Oh," I fumbled. I felt embarrassed. I was still learning the difference between grasping and trying. I wasn't sure if my honesty had come off as an act of confidence or desperation.

He smiled nervously. "I've just seen the end of a relationship."

His phrasing was notably passive, ambiguous. I wondered who broke up with whom.

"Oh," I said. "I'm sorry to hear that."

"I'd like to get together," he said. "At least to have coffee."

"That would be great," I said.

"After grades are turned in," he said.

I sensed his hedging.

"I'm not going to chase after you," I said, pulling back. "If you want to get together, reach out."

"I will," he said, looking me in the eye.

I almost believed him.

He never followed through, and I never saw him again, unless you count almost two years later, when I saw him virtually, when I stumbled upon his online dating profile:

> I'm passionate . . . I give everything to those things worth giving anything to. I'm loyal . . . once you're in the inner circle, I take it very seriously. I'm curious . . . learning is sexy.

He was looking for his match:

> You care about worldly events, love dogs, challenge norms, want to pursue and not just be pursued, value intellectual sparring, work to understand and not just critique, enjoy people watching, recognize complexity in people's character, are self-aware, and think the best moments oftentimes result from a balance of planning and spontaneity.

I felt a wave of longing for the relationship I'd wanted with him. Then I came upon his "stats" column, where he listed his habits and preferences:

> Smoking: Sometimes
> Drinking: Often
> Drugs: Sometimes
> Relationship Type: Mostly monogamous

Jonathan? I read it again to make sure.

I'd dodged a bullet.

Who Knows, Could Be

DURING THE SIX months I went speed dating, on my scorecard I checked off the names of four men: Lou, Leo, Mason, and Corey. Leo and Corey were my "mutual matches." At first, I considered what I'd done to turn off Lou and Mason; I took a critical eye to my self-presentation, deconstructed how I might've appeared, how I'd failed, what I'd said. But then I stopped myself. I managed to let go of my need to achieve the impossible task of eliciting interest.

If he's not into you, he's not for you.

Leo started dating an old flame soon after our speed date and decided not to meet with me. But Corey called and asked me out.

For the record, while I do enjoy four-star treatment, I'm not all that impressed by wealth and elitism. I feel uncouth around designer labels, overpriced food, and expensive décor. So when Corey took me out to dinner at a fancy restaurant in Cambridge, I didn't feel at ease. While another woman might've felt won over, I wasn't.

Handing me a menu, Corey invited me to go home with him—"after we eat, of course," he added—and then proceeded to decide what would be best for me to have for my meal, telling the waiter we'd have the eight-course sampler for two, and then asked me several more times if I'd go home with him.

I wasn't just turned off, I was annoyed, especially when he disclosed that he was still "technically" married.

"My wife doesn't live with me," he assured me. "She's down the street." They were separated. He explained the arrangement was for easy co-parenting of his three kids.

I felt more than bothered by Corey. And yet, I didn't end our date. I didn't get up from the table and leave. Instead, I went with my longtime default—I questioned my perception: What was wrong with me? Corey seemed to think this was all perfectly normal. I wondered, was I looking at the situation through the lens of PTSD or would any woman be put off by such behavior?

I was tired of the way my upbringing still prompted me to question my gut.

Corey said other women he went on dates with didn't think his marriage status was "a problem." Why was it an issue for me?

"I don't date married men," I said.

"It's just a legality," he said. "I don't really understand why you're so upset. I've been married for nineteen years so I'm out of practice when it comes to dating protocol. Would most women react this way?" He sounded genuinely curious.

Did it matter?

Corey had triggered me, and I watched part of myself get caught in the web of my past. I was afraid, not of potentially appearing rude to my date by leaving, but of being so bold by defying social etiquette. I thought the universe might punish me. I was afraid of getting sexually assaulted if I left the restaurant, which was located in a dicey section of town. It was already after dark. I'd have to walk to my car alone. Not to mention, who was going to pay for the $325 meal, an amount equal to almost twenty percent of my monthly income?

When the check came, I went to the ladies' room to breathe, to get grounded. By the time I returned to the table, to my relief Corey had paid. He walked me outside, where I told him I didn't think we were compatible. He begged to differ. He wanted a lover. He wanted one now.

I left, quickly.

———

I dealt with my date with Corey in the way I dealt with much of my life: I wrote about it to make sense of it, to purge it. When the *Huffington Post* published it, I felt a slight twinge of guilt for having made public the details of my date with Corey. I didn't want to be the kind of woman others saw as playing kiss and tell. But I told myself a) we hadn't kissed and b) the situation warranted expression. I hadn't used his name. I hadn't outed him. I'd outed myself, for the first time, without fear, with my uncensored thoughts, my unapologetic voice.

"Public Service Announcement for a First Date"

The following is a public service announcement brought to you by a first date.

On our first date, don't tell me I really must see the 1965 exploitation film *Faster, Pussycat! Kill! Kill!* after I've told you I have a master's degree in screenwriting. It is not going to make me want to see you again, even if you take me out for a $325 dinner consisting of food I cannot pronounce and that is the shape of nickels and dimes, part of which has the texture of a slug. I don't need to have my fork and knife replaced after two bites six times. I don't own that many utensils.

The difference between sparkling and bottled water, only one of which the restaurant will charge us for, does not impress me (neither does your PhD in molecular biochemistry and biophysics from Yale or your fellowship from Harvard or your MBA from MIT, though originally that, along with your good looks, kind smile, interest in hiking and the outdoors, and your work in cancer research made me think you might be a "good catch").

At the start of our date, don't ask me if I'll go home with you after dinner, and don't ask me another six or seven times at fifteen-minute intervals after I've said no, or withhold information about yourself with the promise of divulging it only if I go home with you, and don't ask me to provide a more legitimate reason for not wanting to go home with you. Also, don't say before I agree to our date that you're interested in ultimately finding a long-term relationship, after I've told you that that is my reason for dating, and then on the date say to be honest really now that isn't true.

Don't ask me to believe that you think a man asking a woman to go home with him, or a woman asking a man the same, doesn't mean sex. You've already admitted to knowing backward and forward every Seinfeld episode, including the one where George's date asks him to come up to her place for coffee. Don't tell me that if I go home with you that we'll "just watch a movie."

Don't tell me there's something about my eyes that has made you talk about the details of your sex life with your "ex"-wife and that you hope you haven't over-shared, and don't ask if I've ever considered being a therapist, especially after you've just said you don't really believe in therapy, though you've tried it and it's been helpful. Don't explain that the woman you've spent your life with since college asked you a few months ago at the age of forty-three to try out BDSM, including the use of whips, to save your then "intimacy-less" marriage, unless the point is to share something that could make or break my decision to go on a second date with you.

Don't think about asking me to "go for a walk" in a dangerous neighborhood in the dark after a three-and-a-half-hour dinner after I've said I have to be going now. Don't stall by lecturing me on film history. Don't tell me you read *Brave New World* by choice when you were ten and don't prepare a list of novels you've read that I haven't but must in order to educate myself on "what is good literature." You are a scientist, after all.

Don't force me to make up a story about my cat having a life-threatening medical issue that requires me to go home without further delay and don't think I owe you a kiss because you picked up the check.

Above all, make sure you're actually officially divorced before you ask someone for a date, and don't let the door hit you on the way out.

—Published in the *Huffington Post*,
written by Tracy Strauss

After Corey, I thought it might be time to come to peace with what was to be my life sentence: singlehood. I thought that my dating life was ill fated, and that there was nothing I could do to change its course.

Then something unexpected happened.

I'd just walked in the door after a therapy session, my eyes and cheeks still damp from crying. My mood was low. I was forty years old and single, working one full-time and two part-time teaching jobs, still struggling to make ends meet, though I'd finally been able, using funds from the sale of my mother's condo, to move out of the garret and into a one-bedroom apartment, a unit with a full-sized refrigerator and a living room in which I could actually fit a couch and stand up without hitting my head on the ceiling.

I tossed my keys and purse onto my small entryway table, fed Hannah and Sam their dinner, and then sat down at my desk, in front of my computer, and checked my email. Among several work-related messages and a couple of notes from friends, there was an email from a daytime TV talk show producer. He'd read *Public Service Announcement for a First Date*. He asked if I'd be interested in coming on the show to share my story and get some help with the dating scene.

My heart pounded. I wondered if this was some kind of prank. My old high school insecurities flashed through my mind: I was the nerdy girl the popular crowd made fun of for my unstylish hair, my lack of "cool" clothes, and the fact that I never had a boyfriend. I thought I was the last person a television show would be interested in spotlighting. I checked with my agent, who confirmed: This was no joke; this was legit. It was a respected, "feel-good" show. Did I want to go on television?

Did I? I didn't know. I was a writer, an introvert, the antithesis of a TV personality. In publishing essays about overcoming my past, I had relative control over how I presented myself through written words. Writing gave me a sense of mastery. But television was wrought with unknown variables: vulnerability.

My throat itched with excitement and fear.

Spontaneity, which I imagined was the core requirement of any talk show appearance, wasn't my strength. Look what happened when I let it ride with the hot ginger-haired chef. And remember my "Acting for Non-actors" class, my worst nightmare? But this wouldn't be acting, I told myself. This would be *real*. I'd be myself: a writer and a professor. Yet I understood that the show would probe beyond my professional roles—this was about dating, after all. I was almost certain that they'd uncover some inherent trait that would render me unlikable to the world. I thought about Serena and my therapy group, and my first boyfriend Mitch, and suddenly my old fear resurfaced: My truth would be a turn-off, a deal breaker. And then: I was tired of being afraid.

The invitation was there. Was I interested?

Suddenly, I felt panicked by the prospect of success. And yet, something inside me said, *go for it*. What did I have to lose?

Mr. & Ms. Right

THE *MERRIAM-WEBSTER* DICTIONARY defines "Mr. Right" as "a man who would be the best husband for a particular woman." Other sources describe him as the "ideal romantic partner" or "perfect marriage partner."

I didn't want "perfect." "Perfect," as I'd ascertained from my experience with my former boss, was too much pressure. I didn't trust "perfect." "Perfect" wasn't real. But I was certainly looking for a better man than the men I'd met. I was looking for you. Yet, after so many bad dates, frankly, I wasn't sure you existed. Coupling that with an insecurity that I wasn't, in my own right, "Ms. Right" material, I thought the cards were stacked against me.

In truth, you were out there. But in order to open up my life to the real possibility of finding you, I had to let go of the fear that was stopping me.

———

"I don't know if I can do this!" I burst into tears in Dr. Ross's office the day of my scheduled flight out west, where the talk show was produced.

Writing about my personal life was one thing but coming out from behind my typewritten words and going on a talk show to discuss it was something else. Why did they think I was so special? I heard my mother's distrusting voice saying, *they're going to trick you, don't go, you'll make a fool of yourself, they'll humiliate you on national television.* I felt a bit wary, though I considered that my mother's fears, and my trauma history, might be acting like a camera scrim, tinting my view.

Despite my trepidation, I wanted to do it. A door had opened, and I wanted to walk through it to see what opportunities I might find, and not just in dating. I thought appearing on a television show might boost my career credentials and make me a more competitive candidate in the job market. But I was afraid of exposing myself in an arena that was completely out of my comfort zone.

It was my choice.

"You can change your mind at any time," Dr. Ross said. "Remember that."

We worked on visualization techniques to cope with my phobia of flying, from the stages of airport arrival, to aircraft boarding, takeoff, in-flight time, and landing. Being on a plane, particularly during turbulence, reminded me of being in the car when my father tortured me on the hills of Old Montauk Highway: I lacked control, I couldn't get out, I thought I'd die. Although I logically knew the difference between a car and a plane, the past and the present, my nervous system didn't: I went into panic mode.

But I was afraid of much more than flying. I was terrified of putting myself out there, of truly being seen.

———————

I arrived at Boston's Logan airport after a full day of teaching, with my students' midterm essays packed in my overstuffed luggage. The smell of the airport made me gag. My body started to tremble.

I made it through the security checkpoint and went straight to the ladies' room and locked myself in a stall, shaking and crying silently for a long time, letting out my anxiety. When I heard the boarding announcement for my flight I thought about how easy it would be to not get on the plane, and how disappointed I might feel if I didn't.

I took a deep breath. I gathered my things. I opened the stall door and went to the gate. I got on the plane. I flew out west.

———————

The talk show sent a stretch limo to pick me up at the airport. Inside the limo there was a bar, temperature control and radio station keypads, an intercom, and streaming colored lights. I messaged my friends: *It looks like a disco in here.* They requested I take a selfie and share. I tried not to get motion sick as I angled my camera and posted a photo.

I felt nauseous and tired from traveling, but now I also felt excited.

At the hotel, I checked into my room. I took a muscle relaxant my dentist had prescribed to combat the severe TMJ I'd developed in the days leading up to my trip, and then I went to bed.

The following morning, the first day of taping, I awoke in my hotel room feeling disoriented: Where was I? What was I doing? Although I didn't know it then, my double-episode appearance on the talk show would include a discussion of my dating difficulties, advice from the host, a makeover by a famous fashion expert, lessons with a celebrity confidence coach, and a blind date.

At the studio, I was led from the wardrobe department to the makeup department to the green room, all the while with the head producer beside me, running down the show's agenda to present me as a forty-year-old relationship blogger for *the Huffington Post* "who lacks confidence" in the dating scene. I was nervous about how accurately they'd present me, about how I'd be seen by the world—by people who didn't know me. I couldn't stop my body from shaking. I had trouble retaining information. I was afraid I might blank out in front of the cameras.

I'd wanted to be open to a new experience but now I began to plot my escape. I entertained the idea of leaving the studio before the start of the show, jumping in a taxi and flying back to Boston. Who would notice? I caught myself: I was in "fight or flight" mode.

I was on the verge of a full-blown panic attack when a tall debonair man approached and extended his hand, introducing himself. He said he saw my fear and he understood it. He told me to "own it."

I told myself to take a breath. I reminded myself that I was exhausted and anxious, so my reactions might be heightened. My gut told me to stay, despite my fear. I sensed there was something important that would unfold if I did.

And so I went on set, and I met the host, and I began to discuss my story. And when I smiled and my upper lip got stuck on my front teeth because my mouth was so dry from nervousness, I tried not to worry that the audience would notice.

When the makeover commenced, my curly blonde hair was transformed with dark brown extensions into long, sleek tresses. I was dressed in a new wardrobe, clothing I could never afford on my salary. My face became a canvas for palettes full of makeup. A producer said I looked "like a model, like a Barbie doll."

The audience cheered.

I liked the positive attention, but negative body image issues I'd struggled with years before resurfaced. I thought about how easy it must be for actresses to fall down the slippery slope of eating disorders and plastic surgery.

———————

By the time the segment taping was over, it was evening. I went back to my hotel and called Dr. Ross. We'd planned to have Skype sessions periodically during my days out west. "You may not recognize me," I told him over the phone.

When his face appeared on my computer screen, I started to cry. I'd been compartmentalizing my PTSD so that I could focus on what I needed to do during the show. Now, I let it out.

"Do you regret going?" Dr. Ross asked.

"No," I said, a thick coat of mascara and five layers of eyeliner running down my face. "But it's been challenging."

We talked about ways I could continue to manage my anxiety, and perhaps, even, enjoy the ride.

———————

For part two of the show, a celebrity confidence coach led me through a series of "confidence-boosting exercises," including how to walk with "swag" in five-inch heels. She recommended how to appear confident on a dinner date, how to hold my posture, how to lean in, maintain eye contact, and strategically touch my date's arm—and then she had me practice. I felt awkward and nervous at first, but I was open to trying new things. We made a list of appropriate topics for good first date conversations—pets, careers, the weather, pop culture, working out—and topics to avoid, including sex, dating, politics, and religion. Finally, she had me look in a full-length mirror and write words on it that reflected the person I am.

"Tell yourself you're this guy's dream date," she said. "Because you are."

Finally, it was time to utilize my newly acquired appearance and skills on a blind date. With a microphone taped to my bra, at a fancy steakhouse downtown, I tried to remember all the things my confidence coach had told me to do to appear confident, but I felt so on edge that I could no longer keep any of it straight. Meeting Jake, a forty-two-year-old university administrator, was what I'd been waiting for. I shut my eyes and listened to my inner voice: *Forget everything else. Just be yourself.*

For the first time in my life, I decided it was enough to just be me.

———

The moment we met, my nervousness dissolved. Jake was not only an accomplished professional, but he resembled Paul Walker and Bradley Cooper. He was hot. I felt thrilled. I'd never gone out with a guy who was so good looking. I wondered where he was from (Boston, I hoped), if he was "the one."

Yes, I thought, this all could be worth it.

Five minutes in he asked, "Why are you still single?" At first I thought it was just a line, but he later told me he'd really wondered.

We discovered that we had a lot in common, probably more than the show's host and producers ever knew, including our favorite drink: the Shirley Temple. With his good looks, positive energy, engaging smile, emotional depth, sense of humor, and his passion for his profession, he was so much of the man I'd been looking for in a potential boyfriend but yet hadn't found in all my years of dating.

———

When our TV date was over, Jake asked if I wanted to go somewhere for dessert so that we could get to know each other without the cameras.

At a bakery across town, he treated me to brownies and began to discuss his life. He told me he'd gotten divorced five years earlier. He'd been burned. He said he was firmly anti-marriage and anti-kids. He was looking for a long-term relationship, but "without any strings attached."

"Why?" I asked.

"I need an easy out if things go badly," he stated.

My heart sank. I ultimately wanted marriage and to raise a child. But at my age, were my aims achievable? Should I give up these things? Jake had many of the traits I was looking for in a potential boyfriend and life partner. I thought perhaps I was being unrealistic in wanting more.

When the bakery closed, Jake hailed a taxi and took me back to my hotel, where we chatted for another hour in the lobby. We talked candidly about our lives, about our search for a mate, about going on a TV date. I didn't know anything about Jake before our first date, but he revealed to me that he'd Googled me. He'd read my essays.

"I admire your courage and strength," he said.

He told me he was raised in the Boston area by a psychologically abusive father and an emotionally absent mother. He said he'd had his own struggles, but he'd worked in therapy to overcome them. He'd moved out west after graduate school and had been there ever since. In his free time, he was an instructor for a women's self-defense class. Jake accepted my past and actually saw me in a more positive light because of what I'd done to surmount it.

I felt a fast bond forming between us. I told myself that he might be "the one." I tried to forget that he wasn't looking for marriage and kids. No man was perfect, and, compared to the other men I'd dated, I thought Jake was pretty amazing.

When he asked if I'd like to get together again before I left town, I said yes. It'd been a long while since I'd felt attracted enough to someone to move past Date #1. I was hoping he might take me sightseeing—I was spending the weekend there before the final episode taping—but he had to work, so I went solo, with plans to meet him for dinner.

For decades, my mother had warned me that young women who travel alone get raped, abducted, and killed. She'd seen an incident on the news, which grew global in her mind. She projected onto the world the reality of the home in which I was raised; she saw herself—and by extension, me—as a vulnerable target, a perpetual victim. For so long, I didn't see that she projected onto me all that she couldn't handle. I had a college friend who traveled to the Bahamas by herself, several times. Nothing bad happened to her. But in my mother's mind, and subsequently in mine, venturing out was dangerous

Now, six years later, I wasn't going to allow my mother's persistent voice, which I'd internalized, to prevent me from pursuing opportunities. Although it was tough work to divorce myself from her beliefs, I vowed not to live in her realm of terror and pain.

On my own, I explored the city. I took an architectural boat tour, walked downtown to the art museum, and went to a butterfly sanctuary, where I sat in the peaceful quiet of fluttering wings, taking in how my mother's fears about being a woman traveling alone were unfounded.

On our second dinner date, without an audience, I decided to ask Jake if he'd tell me more about what he meant about needing "an easy out" in a relationship. If I was going to date him, I wanted to understand his stance further: How wedded to the idea was he?

He explained he'd suffered terrible emotional pain at the hands of his ex-wife, who wanted children and had left him because he didn't want to have offspring. "I won't let a woman do that to me again," he said. "I won't wait for a safe to fall on my head."

At first I felt sympathetic, but the more he talked about it, the more I realized he saw every woman he'd dated since his divorce as his ex-wife. He hadn't let go of her. It had been five years since their split, but he still lived in the condo they'd bought and resided in together. I thought it'd be better to move, to leave behind the pain, but Jake disagreed: "I'll lose all the money I put into it if I sell it," he said. In fact, he'd taken on a second job to pay his mortgage and was looking for a third.

The more he talked, the more I saw that Jake's existence revolved around suffering. That's how I perceived it, anyway. He shared how lonely he felt, and how he frequently woke up in the middle of the night from nightmares he didn't recall. He told me he wanted me to be there to hold him; he pictured me comforting him. The more he revealed, the more he sounded as if he was looking for a woman as a salve to his wounds, the key to solving his problems. I was reminded again of the line "You complete me" from *Jerry Maguire*. I wanted to be with someone who was already complete, and who saw me as complete, too.

I knew what I wanted, and what didn't feel right.

"Two of my deepest desires in life are to get married and raise a child," I told Jake. "I want to share my life with a partner and give a child the kind of life I didn't have growing up."

"Those are admirable reasons for marriage and kids," said Jake. "It's just not for me." He explained how he underwent a vasectomy soon after his divorce "so that no woman would try to manipulate or force me into having kids, and then leave me with them," he said. His logic was the opposite of my assumption: I thought most women would take the kids. Jake revealed that the vasectomy procedure had complications and, coupled with two prior hernia operations, he'd suffered "a lot of damage" that could not be fixed. "The vasectomy is *not* reversible," he said adamantly.

"There's adoption," I countered. I knew the reality was it might be too late for me to have a biological child, but I was open to other options. I was curious if any part of Jake was, too. I was also a little disturbed by the extent of the details he'd shared after he'd just met me. I felt as if he'd hit me over the head with it.

He scowled and repeated, "I don't want kids." Case closed, discussion over.

I noticed that my body had become tense and I was having trouble swallowing my dinner. I was fighting my intuition. I was beginning to realize that Jake might not be my future life partner after all. And I didn't want that to be true.

———————

After the final episode wrapped, outside the studio building, Jake asked if he could kiss me. I said yes.

We kissed under a starlit sky.

His mouth was soft but urgent. "Wow," Jake finally said, standing back, taking a breath. "You're an amazing kisser."

I thought it was a line.

"It's no line," he said. "I've kissed a lot of women, but it's never been like this."

"Well, I'm kind of out of practice," I admitted. "It's been a while since I last kissed someone."

"It's been six months for me," Jake said, looking at the pavement, as if he were embarrassed.

"Try six years," I whispered.

His jaw dropped. "That can't be possible." He said, putting his arm around me.

He asked if I wanted a ride back to my hotel. I did, but, realizing I'd forgotten my belongings in the green room, we first went back inside. In the studio lobby, audience members flocked to us, calling me "gorgeous." A few asked to take photographs with us, as if we were celebrities. They told us we were "the perfect couple." We were Mr. and Ms. Right. In the moment, it was all very flattering and exhilarating—I was, for the first time in my life, seen as the pretty, popular girl—but it was also quite bewildering.

"Do you want to make out?" Jake asked as we walked to his car in a nearby parking lot.

I did, though I was aware that I was beginning to feel overwhelmed. When he started driving, I became confused. "I thought you meant in the car," I said.

"No," he said. "I meant the hotel."

"Oh," I said. My mind started to race.

"Is that okay?" he asked.

"Yeah," I said. But my gut told me no. I'd been caught up in the excitement of the show, in the audience's fantasy of us as the perfect couple. My heart was beating wildly. I looked out the window for a few minutes, trying to weed through my PTSD versus my real-time feelings about making out with Jake in my hotel room.

"What's wrong?" Jake asked. "You just got really quiet."

I was surprised, and enamored, by the way he seemed to know me.

I was afraid that, if I had him in my hotel room, I wouldn't be able to get him to leave. "I really want to be with you," I said, which was the truth. "But this has all happened so fast. We barely know each other. I don't feel comfortable with you coming up to my hotel room."

"I wasn't talking about having sex," he said. "I was just talking about making out."

I wasn't sure if I believed him, if he was being honest with himself. I didn't know if I trusted him. I didn't know if I trusted myself—I imagined that if he came up to my hotel room, I might not be able to stop myself from having sex with him. If I didn't think I could stop, how could he?

"I'm okay making out in your car," I said. "But I don't want to go to my hotel room."

"Okay," he said gently. "That's what we'll do then."

He pulled into an alley. We started kissing, touching.

"You have such a great body," he said, running his hands around my waist, up my side to the middle of my back, breathing heavily.

No man I'd dated had ever said that to me. I felt my body respond.

Kissing Jake, I wondered, was he attracted to the real me or the made-up me? My appearance had been altered. Part of me felt as if I was making out in the guise of someone else, that I was false advertising, and that this man I adored was feeling up a Barbie doll, not me. I told him so.

"You're one of the most authentic people I know," he said. "I feel a connection between us, something rare."

I, too, felt a connection, one I'd never felt with anyone before. But I also felt something wasn't quite right. Jake's tongue had become pushy, and he tasted less sweet than he had with our first kiss.

"Are you sure you don't want me to come up to your hotel room?" he asked.

The truth was, I wanted to have sex with him. For the first time in my life, I felt ready to truly give myself over to a man—not just sexually but in the sense of sharing myself with him on many levels and being in his life. But his "easy out" stance lit up my mind like a neon sign. While Jake had used the phrase in relation to marriage, the more we'd talked the more I felt it was also his overall approach to life. He was the first man to fall head-over-heels for me and to see me as separate from my past, but, from my viewpoint, he didn't see me as separate from *his* past.

I knew I couldn't be with someone who was preparing for an ending before we'd ventured a beginning. I was already growing attached. While part of me wished to be fine with a fling, I wasn't. I never had been.

I said goodbye.

———————

Back in my hotel room, alone, I felt so many emotions, and a slight PTSD flare up from making out, compounded by physical and emotional fatigue. It was almost midnight and, with the time difference on the East Coast, I didn't want to disturb anyone by calling, but I felt the need to hear a familiar voice, to get grounded. I texted Dr. Ross, hoping we could chat, but he didn't respond. Aunt Nikki had left me a voicemail message saying she wanted me to call her "no matter how late." I dialed her number. I confessed that Jake had asked to come up to my hotel room and I'd declined. Would other women have done it? I was judging myself. She assured me I did the right thing.

When I got off the phone, I went to the bathroom to remove my layers of makeup and false eyelashes. I gave the glued-on hair extensions a tug, but nothing came loose. I stepped into the shower and wet my head. I pulled on the extensions, hard, then harder, but they remained stuck. I used shampoo and conditioner and Vaseline and tried again. I felt like I was ripping a Band-Aid off my scalp, only many times worse. Chunks of my hair came off with the extensions, row after row after row. Finally, I stepped out of the shower and went over to the bathroom sink. I looked at myself in the mirror, wondering how the world saw the real me.

I draped the hair extensions over the nose of the faucet, as if to give them a burial. I began to weep for the pretenses, for the dream that hadn't become reality, and for the realness I found with Jake only to realize I had to let him go. I knew I couldn't change him, though part of me secretly hoped he'd show up at the airport the next morning to tell me he was going to move to Boston to start a life with me, like the way it happens in the movies.

Looking in the mirror again, I finally, viscerally, embraced the importance of committing to my true self, of living and dating from a place of authenticity. Real beauty, real worth, came from within. True confidence was about self-acceptance: loving who I was, flaws and all, and having the courage to put myself out there, to be seen as I really was, knowing there were no guarantees about what might come my way as a result.

I checked the time. I had four hours before I had to get up to go to the airport to head back to Boston. I put on my pajamas and packed my bags. Utterly exhausted, I went to bed.

As I settled under the covers, I heard a couple in the next room having sex and I thought about Jake. I began to touch myself, imagining he and I were making love. I was with the man I wanted—a man who looked like Jake and acted like him, for the most part, but who had done the psychological work necessary to detach himself enough from his toxic past so that he could be in a healthy relationship.

For the first time in my life, I felt I deserved what my heart wanted.

In the days and weeks following my return to Boston, Jake and I would exchange many emails and phone calls. He'd write:

> *Making out with you was...wow. Very special. And we did it (both the kissing and the decisions about it) the perfect way. It was hot, and I am left with zero regrets and wanting more. And thanks so much for being so honest with me about your hotel room—it really made me feel valued and respected that you were so truthful with me about that. You are a beautiful woman.*

He'd ask to visit. I'd decline. I'd express the many things I loved about him—he was kind, passionate, and handsome. He'd tell me he had trouble receiving such compliments: "These are not words I am used to hearing," he'd say. "I miss you." I missed him, too. I'd tell him I'd found myself falling for him, but that I couldn't handle his "easy out" stance. "Women like you don't fall for me," he'd respond. I'd tell him he could visit only if he found himself wanting the same fundamental aims as I did in a relationship. He didn't. He'd beg me to not let go of the joy we'd felt together. I never would. But I also had to move on. We had no future together.

He called me "Tracy Heartbreaker," though I thought he was the real heartbreaker.

At one point, he shared with me his online dating profile, asking if I had any suggestions. I didn't say so, but I didn't really like the man he described. If I hadn't met him in person but had only been scrolling through profiles, I'd never have picked him as a potential boyfriend. The last line read like a throwback to his ex: "And you have to be nice to me."

For a while, I ruminated about whether I'd made the right decision, if I'd passed up an opportunity for true love. My married writer friend Ashley told me a relationship with Jake would've never worked out: "Your decision to not engage in a fling shows your strength, confidence, and integrity," she said. I thought she was just trying to make me feel better, but she wasn't. She was being honest. While I knew the painful aloneness of the single life, she pointed out from her own experience that it was equally, if not more, painful to be with someone and to be, in so many ways, alone in the relationship.

While I felt sad and disappointed about how things had turned out, in the end I also felt hopeful. My rendezvous with Jake wasn't just some big tease. He embodied elements of the man I was searching for, which made me revel in possibility.

CHAPTER 11

AT LAST

NINE MONTHS AFTER my television stint, I passed a discount shoe store on my way home from The Writers' Room of Boston, where I was their new nonfiction fellow. I'm not a woman who loves to shop, but for some reason I felt compelled to go inside the store.

On the clearance rack, I saw a pair of blue suede four-inch heels, shoes the talk show's wardrobe department had had me try on. They were the only heels that I could walk in without pain. Now they were in front of me, the only pair and in my size. I put them on. I felt like Dorothy in *The Wizard of Oz*, seeing her ruby slippers, finding out that she had the power inside her all along to go where she desired. I imagined the shoes had traveled all the way from out west to find me in Boston. It was fate, kismet, destiny. I bought them.

A week later, I wore my new shoes on a date with a man who seemed to have all the traits I was looking for in a life partner in list form on his online dating profile. I was enthusiastic. For the first time, I felt confident walking in heels. I thought about the show's confidence coach and her lessons, and how certain seeds that were planted during the craziness of my time on television had blossomed in my own way and time.

Travis, my date, stood for ten minutes at the bar, grilling me about my career, as if he were conducting a job interview.

"Are you going to sit down?" I asked.

"In a minute," he said.

When he finally did sit, he drank his beer and spilled his entire life's dramas. When he was done, he asked for the check and walked me out.

I noticed that the urgency I'd once felt, the one that had accompanied me on my dates for years—Is he the one? Is *he*?—had faded. The only thing that interested me on this date was my newfound sense of belonging, in my own skin.

I once imagined I'd take my first vacation when I had my first serious relationship, but the reality was I hadn't yet formed such a connection. I was almost forty-two years old, and single. I'd gotten a late start on life and decided not to wait for "Mr. Right" to appear before allowing myself to truly live.

I embarked on my first-ever pleasure trip, three nights in Bar Harbor, Maine.

I'd been on business trips, but never a personal vacation, an experience I desired. I'd used the excuse that a vacation was a luxury I couldn't afford. But what had really held me back was my mother's ingrained fear: *Women who travel alone get abducted.*

Now my mother was long gone, and I was using money I'd received from her estate settlement to pay for my trip. I was going to unwind, relax.

I arrived on Mount Desert Island safely after a five-hour drive from my apartment. Along the way, I texted my friend Guy. Guy and I met when we were editors on the high school newspaper; I'd asked Guy to be my date to the junior prom, where he was more interested in the fashion of my dress than I was. Now Guy, a gay man and newly single, was living close to me, in Cambridge, where we often met up to trade stories and talk about our hopes and dreams. We frequently texted each other about the trials of online dating:

(Guy) I've been chatting with one buff 49 yr old about Edith Wharton's *Age of Innocence* and the '93 film but he doesn't even have a face picture and I think the chat is pretty much at an end.

(Me) Got a message from someone named "Guyyyyyy" age 49, no pic.

(Guy) It wasn't me, I swear!

(Guy) Ugliest guys write to me on okc. I feel like a troll when I only ever get msgs from ugly 54 yr olds. And it's yet another porno: "am gifted with using it, and pretty awesome at giving head."

(Me)   I think it's time for me to remove my okc profile. My latest message: "Your smile is fascinating that it could devor [sic] a man of God, if you wouldn't mind, I would like to ask you, how was your day?"

(Guy) Starbucks Harvard Sq is the place to be at night! Sitting next to a hot jock lawyer (I think—he's reading Stanford law review) but he also has a wedding band! and now he's reading a Hebrew website. A Jewish jock lawyer—swoon!

(Me)   One of these days we have to hit the jackpot. The pendulum has to swing the other way at some point, right? Isn't that a law of physics?

(Guy) YES.

Guy knew I had PTSD and fears about traveling. Two hours into my drive to Maine, at a rest stop, I texted him for a reality check when I panicked that my apartment might get robbed in my absence: Had I left my bank account information out in the open, along with all my passwords? He texted in response: "It's anxiety. Don't worry. You'll feel better once you get to your destination."

He was right. When I arrived at the B&B, Ben, a nice-looking late thirty-something innkeeper, greeted me.

"It's just you?" he asked, as if I were a rare type of guest.

I felt the need to justify my presence. "Yes," I said, trying to think of a legitimate explanation. "I'm a writer. I'm here to pen the next *Eat, Pray, Love*."

Ben smiled. I blushed.

———

An hour later, I ventured out on a guided sunset sea kayaking tour. I put aside my worry about what the four romantic couples in attendance might think of me, the "plus one" for whom the tour guide had to special-order a single among the tandem kayaks. I didn't want to miss out just because I was solo. Ashley and my other married friend, Kyle, said I was fortunate to be unattached: I could do whatever I wanted whenever I wanted. I was free.

Paddling in a kayak, I marveled at the speed at which two people could travel across water versus one. I pushed through the heavy ocean current as fast and efficiently as I could, following the tour guide's recommendation to utilize my abdominal muscles as well as my arms, but I couldn't keep up with the group. Blisters began to bubble across my palms. My shoulders grew fatigued. A motor-boat roughened the surf. Waves of fear washed over me—*What if I can't do this? What if my mother was right? What if I capsize, or get lost at sea?*

Just keep going, I told myself.

Eventually, the tour guide stopped so that she could highlight facts about the coast, and I caught up. Joining everyone, my anxiety faded. I looked around at the beauty of Frenchman Bay, the Porcupine Islands, and an eagle circling above. I felt myself ease.

Then I got seasick.

As the group paddled onward, I tried to ignore my rising nausea and dizziness, hoping the sensations would go away. But as we continued, I felt worse, and worse.

Forty-five minutes into the two-and-a-half-hour excursion, I politely asked the guide if anyone had ever gotten seasick on her tour.

"On a scale of one to ten, how sick do you feel?" she asked.

"Eight-point-five," I estimated, the motion of my mouth making me gag.

We paddled quickly toward the nearest island so that I could get out of my kayak and regain my equilibrium. The couples remained in their tandems, watching the sun lower and shimmer across the sea. I stepped in the other direction, onto solid ground, walking over to a boulder and sitting down. I was embarrassed and shivering. I vomited and cried.

I tried to console myself: *At least this isn't your honeymoon.*

The sun set.

"I know the last thing you want to do is get back in the kayak," the tour guide began, "but we have to return to shore before dark."

I was too weak to paddle, so she tied my kayak to hers to tow me in. Twenty minutes later, we docked at the harbor. Hyperventilating, I had to be lifted out of the single because my hands had gone numb.

Originally, I'd planned to take myself out to dinner, but now I couldn't consider the idea of food. I walked back to the B&B, where, through the front window, I saw Ben on a couch watching television with his girlfriend, a curly brunette.

I walked into the foyer with my shorts soaking wet.

Ben's cocker spaniel trotted over to me.

"Did you go out to dinner?" Ben asked.

"No," I said, bending down to receive the dog's affection. My head felt heavy. "I went on a kayaking tour. I'm very seasick. I'm going to take a shower and get to bed."

"Alright," said Ben.

"Feel better," said his girlfriend.

———

For years, I'd been afraid of sleeping alone in a hotel room. On business trips, I barricaded the door with a piece of furniture, terrified of a potential intruder, of being raped and killed. But my first night in the B&B, I felt so miserable that the thought never crossed my mind. What I was apprehensive about was whether I might die in my sleep. I felt so sick. Being by myself had its drawbacks: What if I needed help in the middle of the night?

I texted Ashley to ask if she, a mother of three, thought I was okay. Were my electrolytes out of balance? Was I at risk for convulsions?

Ashley understood my fear. She asked if I'd peed, a telltale sign of whether I was dehydrated enough to need medical care. Yes, I just had. She told me I was all right, to just drink as much water as I could and to sleep off the seasickness.

I did.

———

For the rest of my vacation, I stayed on land. I biked and hiked, exploring Acadia National Park. I took several selfies and posted them on Facebook to document my vacation, to share with my friends. I enjoyed myself.

Although I'd missed the sunset while kayaking, I watched it while sitting atop Cadillac Mountain, the highest point along the north Atlantic seaboard. Taking in the vastness of the universe, the sky's deep pink-purple majesty, I felt part of something larger than myself, something sublime. Simultaneously, I keenly felt my separateness, my aloneness. I wanted to reconcile these two states of being.

———

My last evening in town, I had dinner at a restaurant overlooking the harbor. Eating by myself, I thought about my kayaking adventure. I'd had some difficulties but, I pointed out to myself, I hadn't capsized. I hadn't gotten lost at sea.

For years, I'd believed my dating life was all for nothing, but in truth it wasn't—on the way to finding you, I found myself. Now, I took stock of where I'd been, of how far I'd come. For the first time in my life, I liked who I was. I might've even loved myself, too.

I noticed the empty chair across the table. I hoped to one day have a significant other with whom I could share life's journey, but for now one thing was certain: The life partner I'd been searching for had been there all along. That person was smart and resourceful and full of passion. That person was devoted and dependable and true. That person was me.

And then, not too far down the road, to my sheer wonder and delight, I met you.

ACKNOWLEDGMENTS

I COULD WRITE a book thanking every person who's been part of my journey, but I have a two-page limit, so, I send my deepest gratitude to you all, with special thanks:

To my first grade teacher, Ms. Belensky, for fostering my joy and love of storytelling, for asking me over and over, "and then what happened?"

To my graduate writing mentors, who read early drafts of my manuscript and provided critical feedback and guidance: Leah Hager Cohen, Richard Hoffman, Alex Johnson, Rachel Kadish, and Kyoko Mori (and for the love of cats).

To Joseph McCartin, for "American Society Since 1945," for playing that clip from *Rebel Without a Cause*, and for helping me discover my voice. To Rachel Hall, Ron Herzman, Carol Highsaw, Maria Lima, and Gene Stelzig, for your positive and enduring influence on my writing and teaching life. To Steve Konick, for "closer to fine." To Graham Drake, for your faithful encouragement and for always reminding me to "follow your star."

To Henry Dane, Michael Lowenthal, and Darin Strauss for your countless hours of advice. To Kent Wolf, who first believed in the power of my story. To Judy Linden, for your book proposal expertise.

To Kaylie Jones, for filling in for Frank McCourt that summer at the Southampton Writers Conference, for seeing promise in my writing and for telling me to push forward even if I felt afraid. To Stephen Geller, for the program that set me on my writerly course.

To the hardworking staff and faculty at writers conferences that were pivotal to my growth: Bread Loaf Writers' Conference, Norman Mailer Writers Colony, Southampton Writers Conference, Tin House Writers Workshop, and the Wesleyan Writers Conference. To the Writers' Room of Boston, for providing me with the space to write and share my work, for the most accepting community of writers I've ever known, and for the most creative use of a bathroom wall.

To Kate Gilbert for the luck jar and all our runs to Bourbon. To Lynne Anderson, Kathryn Kopple, Evan Roskos, and Louise Tolmie, for our great escape from the pig roast and other middle-of-nowhere corruptions. To Gina Bednarz, for our fortune-cookie lunch at rez.

To May Cobb, for telling me to write that essay and for reminding me, even in the darkest of times, to *believe*. To Luis Alberto Urrea for introducing us in the Cabin, for your inclusivity, and for saying, "don't let the bastards get you down!"

To Lois Glass, Mary Harvey, and the Boston Area Rape Crisis Center, for raising awareness and helping survivors of sexual trauma to heal.

To A. Bokunewicz, for welcoming me into your Zumba class. And to my Zumba students, for being in the room.

To Melissa Faliveno, Meredith Goldstein, Ann Hood, Sue Monk Kidd, Sue William Silverman, and Amanda Stern, for your generosity of spirit. To Marisa Siegel and Mary-Kim Arnold, for the opportunity to serve as essays editor for *The Rumpus*. And to all the writers who sent essays my way, for trusting me with your stories. To the editors who've published my work, especially Sarah Hepola, Kevin Larimer, Tyler Moss, and Jessica Strawser; and to Lou Ann Walker and *The Southampton Review*, for my first major publishing credit. To Laura Gianino, for your advice and camaraderie. To Janeane Bernstein, for having me on your show. To Nile Hawver, for your talented photography. To Kim Gravel, for believing in me.

To Jim Milliot, Louisa Ermelino, and *Publishers Weekly* for printing my story. To Mark Gompertz, for offering to publish my book, making my dream come true. And to Caroline Russomanno, editor extraordinaire, for championing my pages.

To the Barbara Deming Memorial Fund, for providing financial assistance. To the Cambridge Public Library, for the Silent Room, where I spent many hours on this book. To Toni Long and Jonathan Lyons, for your insights. To Dr. Paul Dobrin and his staff, for problem-solving smiles.

To my friends, especially Scott Alessandro, Kara Cilano, Perri Trainer Davis, Linda Mallon Dias, Jodi Yorio Finlayson, Lilach Fisher, Irline François, Nancy Howell, Erin Kemper, Danielle Sicari Newland, Dave Peykar, Michael Stevenson, Kristin Greeley Thompson, and Jennifer Zobair, for being in my life. To Jeff Lieber, for so much but especially for the "big enough book" moment. To Neil A. and Rob B., for inspiration. To Marilyn O'Brien, for taking care of Hannah and Sam in my absence.

To my family, especially Lenny, Luci, Neal, and all the Winegars. To my dear Auntie Moi, I love you more.

To Rick Greene, for opening your door and helping me find my way. To Harley, for being such a good sport with all those selfies. To Amanda Curtin, Amy, Dave, Jeannie, Judith, Mary-Elizabeth, Matthew, and Shep, for embracing change.

And to my future life partner, to whom I dedicate this book.